Managing
Chronic Fatigue Syndrome
and Fibromyalgia:

A Seven-Part Plan

Bruce F. Campbell, Ph.D.

Foreword by Charles Lapp, M.D.

CSH Press
Palo Alto, California

Note/Disclaimer: The materials in this book are offered for informational and educational purposes. They are not intended to substitute for medical care or other professional advice. The author and publisher do not accept legal responsibility for your use of these materials. Consult your physician or other health care provider regarding your symptoms and medical needs.

The CFIDS and Fibromyalgia Self-Help Program
777 San Antonio Road #121
Palo Alto, CA 94303
Email: info@cfidsselfhelp.org
Website: www.cfidsselfhelp.org

ISBN-10: 0-9705267-1-7
ISBN-13: 978-0-9705267-1-7

This book is available at special discounts for bulk purchases. For more information, contact us.

Contents

I
Understand Your Situation

II
Create a Symptom Management Plan

III
Manage Activity

IV
Reduce Stress and Manage Feelings

V
Recast Relationships

VI
Move From Loss to Hope

VII
Learn Self-Management Skills

Foreword

Perhaps you remember the story of the Holy Grail that was purported to have the miraculous power of restoring health for anyone who found and drank from it. Legend has it that King Arthur sought this divine relic and sent his trusted knights to seek it out.

I occasionally lecture on the Holy Grail because the myth parallels what I hear daily in my practice of medicine: patients on a mission to find a miraculous panacea. This is particularly the case for persons with CFS or FM. Humiliated by doctors who don't understand and rejected by a medical system that relegates CFS and FM to "mental disorders," many begin a pilgrimage to find anyone and anything that might help. Like the Knights of the Roundtable, they make perilous journeys, fight battles along the way and overcome numerous challenges. Most end up worn out and frustrated.

There are a few souls who do find a panacea of sorts. Like Galahad, they discover that reaching the goal is less important than the journey itself. These souls discover that when they've seen all the doctors, tried all the drugs, and explored all the alternatives, the most effective treatment for CFS and FM comes from within: they learn to deal with the illness. While medications may palliate the terrible symptoms, these valiant heroes have learned that CFS and FM are best managed with adaptation and lifestyle changes that lead to new meaning and self worth.

When I first discovered Bruce Campbell's book, I knew that I was close to the Grail. For years I had strived for a cure for CFS/FM, but had come to realize that medically I could only treat the symptoms and optimize my patients' health. Time and nature cured the patient, provided he or she could adapt to a new lifestyle. It was Campbell's book that outlined these adaptations. Since that time, I have encouraged virtually all of my patients to read this book and follow Campbell's advice. He has traversed the dark moors of this illness himself, and he teaches firsthand how to slay the invisible dragon of this illness.

There are no known prognostic factors for recovery from CFS or FM, but from years of experience I can tell you two things. First, those who do poorly are generally overwhelmed by depression and a lack of support. Second, those who do extremely well all share a positive attitude and willingness to adapt. They take control of their own lives and develop new meaning and self worth out of the illness process. As Victor Frankl wrote in his 1959 book *Man's Search for Meaning,* we cannot always choose what life gives, but we can choose how to respond to it.

Most authorities on CFS and FM agree that there are four steps that predictably lead to improvement in CFS and FM. These are:

1. **Symptom management**. Treat symptoms such as pain and sleep disruption that exacerbate and perpetuate the illness.
2. **Pacing**. Ensure rest periods and set reasonable limits on daily activities.
3. **Counseling**. Address depressed mood, anxiety, and emotional stresses; and learn effective coping skills.
4. **Activity**. Take regular low level aerobic exercise.

The book in your hands is a practical self-help guide organized into individual lessons that one can read, assimilate, and put into practice on a regular basis, say one chapter per week. It will walk you step-by-step through the process of adapting to this illness.

Your doctors can help with symptom management and counseling. This volume can guide you through the rest. This book offers hope to those with CFS/ME and FM. There may be no known cure for these conditions, but the book in your hands makes it clear that there are many means to improving quality of life.

Charles W. Lapp, M.D.
Director, Hunter-Hopkins Center
Assistant Consulting Professor, Duke University Medical Center
March 1, 2010
Charlotte, North Carolina

Introduction

This book is the text for the CFIDS and Fibromyalgia Self-Help course, which began shortly after I was diagnosed with Chronic Fatigue Syndrome. I was inspired to create the class by my prior experience at the Stanford University Medical School. Before becoming ill, I had the privilege of working as a consultant to medical self-help programs and saw people gain some control over other chronic illnesses by using self-help strategies like those described in this book. I believed that a self-help approach would also be useful for people with CFS and fibromyalgia. Since our beginnings in 1998, several thousand people from around the world have taken our introductory course and our two additional classes: Creating Your Plan and Living Your Plan.

As our program developed, I made use of the strategies and techniques you'll find here and my health improved. The pace was slow but steady, one or two percent a month over a period of four years. From a starting point of about 25% of normal, I eventually recovered to my pre-illness level of health. (You can read my story at *www.recoveryfromcfs.org*.)

The approach you will find in this book is based on several beliefs:

- People with CFS and FM can find things to help them feel better. These strategies are not aimed at curing either condition, but they can help reduce suffering, improve quality of life and, often, increase functionality.

- A plan for managing CFS or fibromyalgia needs to be individualized for each person's unique circumstances. Your case may be more or less severe than another person's. Also, a person's ability to manage their condition is affected by other factors, such as finances and family situation.

- Long-term illness affects many parts of life, so managing it means much more than treating symptoms. A person also has to address challenges such as controlling stress, managing emotions, building support and finding meaning in a situation of loss.

There are no magic pills for CFS or fibromyalgia. Most experts agree with the idea presented by Dr. Lapp in the Foreword that the most powerful treatment for both conditions is lifestyle change, which means changing our habits and how we live our daily lives. This is a gradual process, changing one or two parts of our lives at a time, but over time it can be transforming. One person in our program, remembering my rate of improvement, calls it the 1% solution.

We have seen many people in our program improve by 20% to 50%, sometimes even more. (You can read about some of them in the Success Stories section of our website: *www.cfidsselfhelp.org*.) In our experience, the keys to improvement are a willingness to adapt and consistent use of the tools of self-management, especially pacing and stress management.

Living with CFS and/or fibromyalgia can feel overwhelming at times. An effective response is to take a series of small steps to regain control. I hope you find in this book ideas for creating *your* 1% solution.

Bruce Campbell, Ph.D.
Executive Director, CFIDS and Fibromyalgia Self-Help Program
March 1, 2010
Palo Alto, California

Understand Your Situation

1. Chronic Fatigue Syndrome and Fibromyalgia

When you develop a long-term condition like Chronic Fatigue Syndrome or fibromyalgia, you may feel like you have entered a new world in which all the rules of life have changed and there is no obvious way forward. This perplexing situation can make you feel helpless. But there are many things you can do to regain control and improve your well being. This book will show you how. Using the ideas you'll find here, you can create a plan for managing CFS and/or fibromyalgia.

The first step, Part 1 in the book, is to understand your situation. We will begin by looking at three key aspects of CFS and fibromyalgia.

Perhaps when you first became ill with CFS or fibromyalgia, you thought you had a short-term illness, but one that kept hanging on. At some point, however, you realized that you had entered a new realm. You were confronted by the fact that your problem was something quite different from a short-term illness. Short-term or acute illnesses are temporary problems that usually end because of medical treatment or the passage of time.

CFS and FM do not create a temporary interruption of your life. Rather, they are conditions that persist. Instead of resuming your previous life after a brief interruption, you were faced with having to adjust to long-term symptoms and limitations. And, if you are like many people with CFS and fibromyalgia, your condition became a focus around which much of your life was oriented. You may also have found that the strategies you use for acute illness, such as pushing through in spite of symptoms, only makes things worse. This book will teach you skills for managing a different kind of illness.

Second, not only do CFS and fibromyalgia impose limits and bring symptoms that persist, they have comprehensive effects, touching many parts of life. They affect your ability to work, your relationships, your moods, your hopes and dreams for the future, and even your sense of who you are. Living with a long-term condition like CFS or fibromyalgia means much more than managing symptoms.

Complicating the challenge, there is an interaction between CFS or fibromyalgia and other parts of your life. (See diagram.) For example, CFS and FM reduce your activity level (arrow pointing out from CFS/FM to Activity), but if you try to do more than your body can tolerate, you will experience higher symptoms (arrow pointing in).

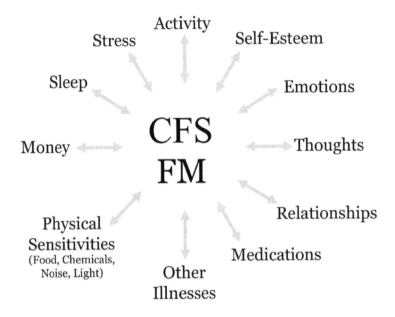

Interactions of illness and other factors

The same pattern of reciprocal effects is true for stress. Living with symptoms on a daily basis is inherently stressful. In addition, illness often creates financial pressures, complicates relationships and brings great uncertainty about the future. In all these ways, illness increases stress. But stress, in turn, can make symptoms worse. Even moderate amounts of stress can greatly intensify symptoms.

Another example is the interaction of illness and feelings. Emotions like worry, anger, depression and grief are normal and understandable reactions to the disruptions and uncertainty brought by serious illness. These reactions to being ill may be particularly intense in CFS and fibromyalgia, because the two conditions make emotions stronger than before and harder to control.

The strength of emotions can create a vicious cycle in which illness intensifies emotions and then emotions, in turn, intensify symptoms. For example, people who are depressed have a lower threshold for pain. Also, pain can be intensified by anger, because anger usually creates muscle tension. Intensified symptoms, in turn, may generate more worry and pessimism.

There are similar two-way interactions between illness and relationships, and illness and money. When someone is ill for an extended period, relationships often suffer because the person who is ill feels discomfort and has less energy, and because others have their lives disrupted, too. But relationship problems, like not feeling understood or worry about being abandoned, create new stresses, that in turn make symptoms worse. Illness affects finances by reducing income. Financial worries then increase stress, which translates into higher symptoms.

To summarize, CFS and fibromyalgia have comprehensive effects, touching many parts of life. They are much more than simple medical problems. A plan for managing them has to address all its effects, not just symptoms.

Third (and perhaps most important), Chronic Fatigue Syndrome and fibromyalgia are affected by how you respond to them. One example is how you live with the limits imposed by illness. One common response is the push/crash syndrome, in which you swing between times of intense symptoms and periods of rest. When symptoms are intense, you go to bed. When they subside, you resume your activity level, but then experience increased symptoms and retreat to bed again. As you'll see in Part 3, pacing offers an alternative. Using pacing, you can replace push and crash with a more stable and predictable life.

While there is so far no cure for either CFS or fibromyalgia, the way a person responds to either condition has a big effect on symptoms and quality of life, often a larger effect than medical treatments. As Dr. Charles Lapp says, "There are limits to what your doctor can do." The key to recovery with these conditions, he says, "is acceptance of the illness and adaptation to it by means of lifestyle changes, for which medical treatment is no substitute."

The self-management approach you'll find in this book provides tools for coping that can also promote improvement and even recovery in some cases. The upcoming chapters contain many ideas for things you can do to feel better. These strategies can help reduce pain and discomfort, bring greater stability, lessen suffering, and may produce improvement, as we have seen many times in our classes.

2. Your Unique Circumstances

Each person with CFS or fibromyalgia is different, so a self-management plan for CFS or FM has to be individualized to fit each person. You can begin to understand *your* unique situation by answering the following questions.

How Severe is Your CFS or FM?

The severity of CFS and FM varies greatly. People's activity level is commonly reduced by 50% to 75%, but the range is wide. Some people are able to continue working, while others have their lives disrupted moderately and still others are housebound or even bedbound. Patterns of symptoms vary, too. Some people may have pain as their major complaint, while for others the main problem is fatigue, brain fog or poor sleep.

Adding to the complexity, each person's illness may vary over time. Some symptoms may disappear, only to be replaced by new ones. Some people may have a relatively stable course, while others may fluctuate between times of severe symptoms and times of remission.

To get an idea of your version of CFS or FM, place yourself on the CFS/Fibromyalgia Rating Scale. If there is a discrepancy between your score based on activity level and your score based on symptoms, rate yourself using the severity of your symptoms. Most people in our program rate themselves between 25 and 45 at the start of the course, but we have had people across almost the full range of the scale.

Your rating gives you an idea of the severity of your illness and the activity level your body can tolerate at the present time. For example, if you rate yourself at 35 (average for people in our program), you can be active about three hours a day without intensifying your symptoms. If your rating is lower, the activity level your body can tolerate currently is likely to be lower. If your rating is higher, you can be more active.

CFS/Fibromyalgia Rating Scale

100 Fully recovered. Normal activity level with no symptoms.

90 Normal activity level with mild symptoms at times.

80 Near normal activity level with some symptoms

70 Able to work full time but with difficulty. Mostly mild symptoms.

60 Able to do about 6-7 hours of work a day. Mostly mild to moderate symptoms.

50 Able to do about 4-5 hours a day of work or similar activity at home. Daily rests required. Symptoms mostly moderate.

40 Able to leave house every day. Moderate symptoms on average. Able to do about 3-4 hours a day of work or activity like housework, shopping, using computer.

30 Able to leave house several times a week. Moderate to severe symptoms much of the time. Able to do about 2 hours a day of work at home or activity like housework, shopping, using computer.

20 Able to leave house once or twice a week. Moderate to severe symptoms. Able to concentrate for 1 hour or less per day.

10 Mostly bedridden. Severe symptoms.

0 Bedridden constantly. Unable to care for self.

Do You Have Other Medical Problems?

Living with CFS or fibromyalgia is often complicated by the presence of one or more additional medical issues. Many people have both CFS and FM. Also, CFS and fibromyalgia are often accompanied by one or more related conditions. In addition, people with CFS and FM often experience conditions common to aging, such as arthritis, back and spinal problems, and high blood pressure.

Here are some of the more common conditions that often accompany CFS and fibromyalgia, listed alphabetically. Most of these conditions are treatable. If one or more applies to you, you can reduce your overall symptom level by addressing them.

- Chemical sensitivity
- Depression
- Food and digestive issues: Candida (yeast infection), Celiac disease, lactose intolerance
- Gastroesophageal reflux disease (GERD)
- Irritable bladder syndrome (interstitial cystitis)
- Irritable bowel syndrome (IBS)
- Lupus
- Lyme disease
- Migraine headaches
- Myofascial pain syndrome (MPS)
- Orthostatic problems such as neurally mediated hypotension (NMH) or postural orthostatic tachycardia syndrome (POTS)
- Restless legs syndrome (RLS)
- Sleep apnea
- Temporomandibular joint disorder (TMJ)
- Thyroid problems

What is Your Life Situation?

Just as people with CFS and fibromyalgia differ in the severity of their illness and their additional medical conditions, so do they come from many different life situations. Some are young; many are middle-aged; some are older. Some are married, while others are single. Some are raising children, while others are empty-nesters. Some are in supportive relationships; others in conflicted ones. Some are financially secure, while others are struggling.

To understand your situation requires that you assess how your unique life situation affects your illness, especially in the areas of resources and relationships.

Some people with CFS or fibromyalgia find their financial situations have changed little since they became ill. Perhaps they have a mild case of CFS or fibromyalgia and can continue to work. Or maybe they have family members who work or they receive disability payments that replace some of their former income. For others, however, financial pressures can be great. Some people live alone with little or no income and no financial cushion. Many are somewhere in between, stressed to some degree, but able to maintain a lifestyle more or less similar to the one they had before becoming ill.

Chronic illness changes relationships, creating new obligations and also new strains and frustrations. You may be single and struggle alone with your illness. Even if you live with a family, you may feel isolated and not understood. All family members are challenged to live differently; some may have to assume additional responsibilities. Relationships can be great sources of support, sources of stress or both.

Your challenges and the resources you have to deal with them will vary depending on your situation. We suggest that to understand your life situation you focus on your family circumstances (single or married, stage in life), your responsibilities (who is dependent on you: often children, sometimes parents, spouse, grandchildren or others), your finances and your sources of support (family, friends, church or other religious group, etc.).

How About Your Coping Skills and Attitude?

Your situation includes two other significant factors: your coping skills and attitude, both of which can be changed. You may not be able to alter the fact that you have CFS or fibromyalgia, but you can learn new and more effective ways to deal with them.

Research has shown that people with chronic conditions can learn effective coping skills through brief self-help classes such as ours. One such program is the Arthritis Self-Help course, which was developed at Stanford University in the late 1970's and has now been taken by over 350,000 people. Participants in the class have significantly reduced their pain and depression, and increased their activity level.

Similar programs at UCLA and Harvard for skin cancer and chronic pain have produced comparable results. People who took a six-session course on coping with skin cancer showed an increase in life expectancy compared to other skin cancer patients. And people who took a course on combating chronic pain reduced their visits to doctors, their levels of anxiety and depression, and their experience of pain.

Using lifestyle changes such as a low-fat diet, exercise and group support, the patients in Dean Ornish's program reversed symptoms of heart disease. In other research, people with diabetes have been able to reduce by half their risk of heart attacks and strokes by improving their regimen of blood testing and insulin injections.

People who improve the most in this type of program are those who believe in their ability to exercise some control over their illness. These people do not deny they are sick or hold unrealistic hopes for recovery, but they have confidence that they can find things to make their lives better. These classes demonstrate that good coping skills can make a significant difference to quality of life and may even change the course of long-term conditions.

Attitude is also important to living well with long-term illness. The attitude that seems to help is one that is both realistic and hopeful. We call it *acceptance with a fighting spirit*. People with this attitude combine two seemingly contradictory ideas. On the one hand, they accept that their illness is a long-term condition. They don't expect a miracle cure to restore them to health. Rather, they acknowledge that their lives have changed and that they have to live differently than before. And they have the conviction that they can find ways to get better through their own efforts. (For some examples, see the Success Stories section of our website: *www.cfidsselfhelp.org*.)

As with other life problems, learning to manage chronic illness involves adapting to new circumstances by making adjustments to daily habits and routines. The upcoming chapters contain many ideas for things you can do to feel better. These strategies are not aimed at curing CFS or fibromyalgia, but they can help improve quality of life and may help you to increase your functional level.

Self-management of long-term illness requires hard work and patience. I hope you can join the many people in our program who have found that they can affect their symptom level and quality of life significantly by accepting responsibility for those things under their control.

PART 2

Create a Symptom Management Plan

3. Symptoms of CFS and Fibromyalgia

Even though there is so far no cure for either CFS or fibromyalgia, there are many ways to alleviate the symptoms of the two conditions. While treatments don't heal either CFS or FM, they can reduce the effects of symptoms and improve quality of life.

The next four chapters describe the major treatment options for the most prominent symptoms of CFS and fibromyalgia: pain, fatigue, poor sleep and cognitive problems. This chapter outlines an overall approach to symptom management. The following four chapters discuss the four main symptoms, beginning with sleep. We start with sleep because poor sleep has such widespread effects and because treating it can improve quality of life and reduce other symptoms.

Before doing that, however, let me add that even though we will focus on four symptoms, people with CFS or FM usually experience several or even many additional symptoms. Other common symptoms in CFS and fibromyalgia include:

- Abdominal pain (bloating, diarrhea/constipation)
- Alcohol intolerance
- Allergies & rashes
- Anxiety
- Chills or night sweats
- Depression
- Dizziness
- Fever
- Headaches
- Jaw pain
- Loss of libido
- Lymph node tenderness
- Nausea
- Numbness or tingling in hands, arms, legs, feet or face
- Ringing in the ears

- Sensitivity to light, sound, smell or weather
- Sore throat
- Weight gain or loss

It also bears repeating that people with CFS and FM often have additional medical problems, so some of your symptoms may be due to other conditions, such as those mentioned in Chapter 2.

Treatment Principles

Managing the symptoms of CFS and FM usually involves the following four principles:

1. **Focus on Improving Quality of Life:** Because so far there is no cure for either CFS or fibromyalgia, the goal of treatment is not healing but rather controlling symptoms and improving quality of life. Medical treatments usually focus on addressing the most bothersome symptoms, such as poor sleep and pain. Self-help strategies like pacing, exercise and stress reduction can also help you feel better and more in control. While treatments don't heal either CFS or FM, they can reduce pain and discomfort, bring greater stability and lessen suffering. They may also increase functional level.

    Treatment of CFS and FM is not limited to addressing symptoms. The two conditions affect many parts of life: people's ability to work, their finances, their relationships, their moods, and their hopes and dreams for the future. Managing them involves much more than just treating symptoms. A self-management plan includes addressing stress and emotions, getting support and recasting relationships, and coming to terms with loss.

2. **Use of Multiple Strategies:** Because people with CFS and fibromyalgia have several to many symptoms and because each symptom may have more than one cause, treatment plans usually involve multiple strategies. For example, treating pain often involves both the use of medications and lifestyle strategies such as improving sleep, pacing, exercise, relaxation, and the use of heat and cold. Cognitive problems ("brain fog") are typically addressed with a variety of techniques, such as the use of lists, pacing, doing one thing at a time, keeping an orderly house, doing mental tasks when sharpest, managing stress, and reassuring self-talk.

3. **Experimentation:** Finding the most helpful combination of treatments often requires experimentation. There is no standard medical treatment for either illness, that is, no medication that is predictably effective. For this reason,

symptom control is usually achieved by trial and error. Experimentation is also useful to find lifestyle adjustments that are effective. For example, you may have to try different exercise programs to find one that helps you without intensifying your symptoms. We call this process of trying different approaches to find what works being your own CFS/FM scientist.

4. Central Place of Lifestyle Change: The things you do and the way you live have a big effect on your symptoms, reducing them if you honor your body's needs or intensifying them if you don't. These impacts are so great that your success in reducing symptoms and regaining control of your life will probably depend more upon your efforts and willingness to adapt to CFS and/or FM than on anything a doctor does for you.

In the words of CFS/FM physician Dr. Charles Lapp, "While your doctor's role is important, you should recognize that there is no known cure for CFS/ME, so there are limits to what your doctor can do." The key to recovery is "acceptance of the illness and adaptation to it by means of lifestyle changes, for which medical treatment is no substitute."

The major symptoms of CFS and FM have several causes in common: overexertion, deconditioning, stress and emotions. Treating these causes with pacing, exercise, relaxation and managing emotions has a multiplied effect, since each strategy affects more than one symptom.

4. Treating Sleep

Poor sleep is an almost universal problem for people with CFS and fibromyalgia. Sleep problems include difficulty getting to sleep, waking in the middle of the night or early in the morning, and over sleeping. Regardless of the number of hours slept, sleep is usually not restorative, meaning that people wake up tired rather than refreshed. In addition to sleep problems due to CFS and FM, a majority of people with the two conditions experience sleep disorders such as sleep apnea and restless legs syndrome.

Addressing sleep problems can be good initial focus for symptom management because treating sleep can both improve quality of life and reduce other symptoms. If you are troubled by poor sleep, consider creating a sleep management plan using a combination of strategies selected from the three approaches described below: improved sleep hygiene, use of medications and treatment of sleep disorders.

Sleep Hygiene: Sleep Environment and Habits

Sleep can be disturbed by such things as irregular hours, a noisy environment, tension and worry, an uncomfortable bed or a noisy sleeping partner. A starting point for better sleep is to address these and other aspects of your sleep hygiene.

1. **Have a Comfortable Environment.** Provide yourself with an environment conducive to good sleep by using a good mattress, and by exercising control over light, noise and temperature. (Note: Noise includes snoring by your sleep partner. Some people with CFS or FM sleep in a separate bedroom from their partner.)

2. **Establish a Routine.** Go through the same routine each night and have a consistent bedtime. Prepare for sleep by gradually reducing your activity level in the several hours before bedtime and by having a regular routine you go through consistently at the same time each night. Your routine might include things like getting off the computer and turning off the TV at a certain hour,

taking a bath, brushing your teeth and reading. These habits can help you wind down and get ready psychologically for sleep.

3. Use Relaxation and Distraction. If you find it difficult to fall asleep, consider listening to quiet music or distracting yourself in some other way, such as by counting or watching your breath.

4. Control Stress and Worry. Stress often leads to muscle tension, which makes falling asleep more difficult. Practicing relaxation methods can help you ease tense muscles. Try relaxation procedures (you'll find examples in articles on our website: *www.cfidsselfhelp.org*) or soak in a hot tub or bath before going to bed.

If you have difficulty falling asleep because you are preoccupied with problems, consider setting aside a "worry time" each night before going to bed. Write down all your worries and what you'll do about them. If worries come up as you are trying to go to sleep, tell yourself "I've dealt with that. I don't have to worry because I know what I'm going to do." Alternatively, you can make an appointment with yourself to deal with the issues the next day, then tell yourself "I've set aside time to deal with that tomorrow."

5. Get Up at the Same Time. If you are going to bed later and later, setting an alarm so that you get up at the same time each day can help you adjust gradually back to more normal hours. Usually, you may not need to compensate by changing your bed time to an earlier hour; your body can adjust itself.

6. Use Pacing. Being too active during the day or early evening can create a sense of restlessness called feeling "tired but wired." Keeping activity within limits and having a winding down period before going to bed are antidotes.

7. Limit Daytime Napping. Often, daytime napping interferes with night time sleep. If you nap during and day and find that you have trouble falling asleep, or your sleep is worse than usual when you nap, you might consider sleeping only at night. (On the other hand, if napping does not disturb your nighttime sleep, you may need more rest.)

8. Avoid Caffeine, Alcohol & Tobacco. Consuming too much caffeine, drinking alcohol and smoking can make getting good rest more difficult. Avoid products with caffeine, such as coffee, tea, soft drinks and chocolate, for several hours before going to bed. Avoid alcohol before bedtime; it can create restless and uneven sleep. The nicotine in tobacco is a stimulant, thus smoking is a barrier to falling asleep.

Medications

Treating sleep with drugs is challenging because there is no single medication that has proven helpful in solving sleep problems for people with CFS and fibromyalgia. Also, many patients develop drug tolerance, so that a medication becomes less effective over time. For both these reasons, sleep problems can benefit from a flexible, experimental approach that utilizes a variety of strategies.

If you think medications might improve your sleep, you might start with non-prescription substances. These include over the counter products like melatonin and valerian, antihistamines such as Benadryl and Tylenol PM. If you prefer prescription medications, a reasonable approach is to find a physician willing to work with you to find what helps in your unique situation. Often a combination of two drugs is prescribed, one to initiate sleep and another to maintain sleep. Medications commonly prescribed to treat sleep problems include zaleplon (Sonata) and eszopiclone (Lunesta) to help you fall asleep and drugs such as cyclobenzaprine (Flexeril), tizanidine (Zanaflex), doxepin elixir, amitriptyline (Elavil) or trazadone (Desyrel) to help you stay asleep.

While medications can improve sleep, they can also make it worse. Some sleep medications that are effective when used occasionally can produce poor sleep if used frequently. Also, some drugs produce side effects, like a feeling of grogginess in the morning. Medications taken for other problems may interfere with sleep if they contain substances like antihistamines or caffeine.

Treating Sleep Disorders

A majority of people with CFS and FM have one or more sleep disorders. Treating them can have a dramatic effect on symptoms. If improving sleep hygiene and using medications don't produce an improvement in your sleep, consider asking your doctor for a referral to a sleep specialist, who can examine you for sleep disorders. Two of the most common disorders are sleep apnea and restless legs syndrome.

Sleep apnea, meaning absence of breathing, occurs when a person's airway becomes blocked during sleep and he or she stops breathing. An episode can last from a few seconds to a few minutes. The person then awakens, gasps for air and falls asleep again, usually without being aware of the problem. The cycle can occur many times a night, leaving the person exhausted in the morning. Sleep apnea deepens the fatigue experienced by people with CFS and fibromyalgia.

Apnea is a treatable condition. A common remedy is the use of a CPAP (continuous positive airway pressure) machine. The patient wears a mask through which a compressor delivers a continuous stream of air, keeping the airway open and thus allowing uninterrupted sleep. Use of a CPAP machine can eliminate 90%

to 100% of a person's sleep apnea. Other treatments are also used for this condition. If you are excessively tired in the morning or have trouble staying awake during the day, you may have apnea.

Restless legs syndrome (RLS) involves "twitchy limbs," strong unpleasant sensations in the leg muscles that create an urge to move. The problem is often at its worst at night. Self-management techniques that may help include reducing consumption of caffeine and other stimulants, establishing a regular sleep pattern, doing exercise that involves the legs, distracting yourself by immersing yourself in activity, using hot or cold baths or showers, and taking supplements to counteract deficiencies in iron, folate and magnesium. Several categories of medications may also help, including sedatives, drugs affecting dopamine, pain relievers and anticonvulsants. Two of the more commonly used drugs for RLS are Requip and Mirapex.

5. Strategies for Pain

Pain is usually the central symptom in fibromyalgia and is often a problem for CFS patients as well. For people with FM, pain is generally felt all over the body, though it can start in one region and spread or move from one area to another. It may be accompanied by neurological problems such as tingling and burning or numbness in the hands, arms, feet, legs or face. For people with CFS, pain may be experienced in the joints or, more commonly, as an overall body pain ("I feel like I've been run over by a truck.")

Because pain in CFS and FM can have a variety of causes, it is usually managed with a variety of strategies. If pain is a problem for you, you can create a pain management plan from the following options.

Medications

People with FM and CFS often treat pain with medications. Because no medication is consistently helpful and because sometimes pain relievers lose effectiveness as the body becomes accustomed to them, experimentation is usually required. Usually, patients begin on dosages that are a small fraction of normal dosage levels.

FM and CFS patients who seek pain relief through medications usually begin with non-prescription products, such as aspirin and other over-the-counter pain relievers. Others find help through prescription medications such as Ultram (Tramadol) and, in some cases, narcotics. Prescription drugs that improve sleep can have a beneficial effect on pain as well. Anti-depressants, such as Elavil (Amitriptyline), Prozac and Paxil are often tried. The FDA (US government body regulating food and drugs) has approved three drugs for the treatment of fibromyalgia: Lyrica (pregabalin), Cymbalta (duloxetine hydrochloride) and Savella (milnacipran HCl).

Many fibromyalgia patients also experience Myofascial Pain Syndrome (MPS), a pain condition localized in trigger points (specific locations in muscles or fascia), often in the neck or shoulders. MPS may be treated with medication and the injection of local anesthetics into the trigger points.

Some patients experience neuropathic or nerve pain, burning or electric shock sensations, felt most commonly in the hands and feet. This type of pain is often treated with anti-seizure medications, such as Neurontin.

Exercise, Posture & Movement

Exercise is one of the most-commonly prescribed treatments for FM and can be helpful for CFS as well. An exercise program done regularly can help reduce stiffness, counteract deconditioning and improve outlook. A program of gentle stretching can be helpful for both FM and CFS. In addition, people with FM are usually helped by frequent breaks for stretching, to reduce stiffness.

FM patients especially can help reduce their pain by experimenting with how they hold their body and how they move. Many patients find that staying in one position for an extended period of time increases stiffness and intensifies pain, so moving periodically can help you avoid pain. Limiting the length of time spent doing repetitive motions like chopping can help, too. For more on exercise and movement, see Chapter 16.

Pacing

A frequent cause of pain is overdoing or having an activity level that is beyond a person's limits. Pacing offers a way to bring stability and control. Pacing can involve a variety of strategies, including:

- Reducing overall activity level
- Setting priorities and delegating
- Taking scheduled rests
- Having short activity periods
- Switching between high and low intensity tasks
- Using the best hours of day for the most demanding activities
- Knowing mental and social limits
- Keeping records to see links between activity and symptoms

For a discussion of pacing strategies, see Chapter 9.

Relaxation

Being in pain can create muscle tension and anxiety, both of which can intensify the experience of pain. Muscle tension is directly painful, while anxiety contributes to the experience of pain indirectly by increasing stress and a sense of helplessness.

Relaxation is an antidote to both tension and stress. Also, it offers a distraction from pain. For some people, relaxation involves the regular use of a formal relaxation or meditation procedure, such as those described in the predecessor to this book, available in the Online Books section at *www.cfidsselfhelp.org*. Other relaxing activities include exercise, mindful breathing, baths and hot tubs, massage, rest breaks and listening to tapes.

Addressing Worry, Frustration & Depression

The experience of pain is intensified by emotions like worry, frustration and depression. Worry and frustration create muscle tension, which makes pain more intense. Relaxation procedures can reduce pain both directly by easing muscle tension and indirectly through reducing stress. People who are depressed have a lower threshold for pain. Self-help strategies, sometimes in combination with medications, can help manage it. For more on feelings, see Chapter 19.

Treating Fatigue & Poor Sleep

Pain, fatigue and poor sleep are tightly connected. Fatigue deepens the experience of pain. When we feel tired, we experience pain more intensely, thus reducing fatigue lessens pain. Similarly, poor sleep intensifies pain, so improving sleep can help control pain. Of the three symptoms, poor sleep is often addressed first.

Heat, Cold & Massage

Heat, cold and massage can be used for temporary relief of pain. Heat is best utilized for reducing the pain that results from muscle tension and inactivity. The warmth increases blood flow and thereby produces some relaxation, reducing pain and stiffness. For localized pain, heating pads or hot packs are used frequently. For overall relief, people often use warm baths, soaks in a hot tub or lying on an electric mattress pad.

Cold treatments decrease inflammation by reducing blood flow to an area. They also may numb the areas that are sending pain signals. You might use gel packs, ice packs or bags of frozen vegetables. With both heat and cold, you should not use the treatment for more than 15 or 20 minutes at a time.

Massage of painful areas can also provide temporary relief from pain. Like heat, massage increases blood flow and can also relieve spasms. You can consider three different forms of massage: self-massage using your hands, massage using a handheld device, and professional massage. If you use a massage therapist, ask her to be cautious and to check frequently on your pain sensitivity.

Problem Solving

You can gain some control over pain by identifying the situations that trigger or intensify pain and then taking steps to change them. For example, you might find that you are not able to keep up with household chores as you used to. Using problem solving, you brainstorm a variety of solutions, such as spreading the chores out over several days, doing them on one day but taking rest breaks, and getting help from others, either family members or hired help. You then try a solution to see whether it works, evaluate and try again.

If you have a job and find that your pain increases when you work under deadlines, problem solving could take several forms. You may train yourself to take time to relax your muscles. Looking at your situation more broadly, you may identify work overload as a recurring problem and consider reducing your hours, changing your responsibilities or taking time off from work. For more on job options, see Chapter 15.

Pleasurable Thoughts and Activities (Distraction)

Immersing yourself in pleasant thoughts and activities can lessen pain by providing distraction. Imagery can be especially helpful, as you visualize a pleasant scene, involving as many senses as possible. If you want to transport yourself to the beach, see the light shimmering on the water, feel the warmth of the sun on your skin, hear the waves crashing and smell the mustard from the hotdogs. Engaging in activities that bring pleasure can also provide distraction from pain. Examples include reading a book, watching a movie, taking a bath, listening to or playing music and spending time in nature.

Healthy Self-Talk

Thoughts can have a dramatic effect on our moods and, in turn, on our perceptions of pain. This can be a vicious cycle. An increase in symptoms may trigger negative thoughts like "I'll never get better" or "It's hopeless." Such thoughts can then make us feel anxious, sad, angry and helpless, intensifying pain and triggering another round of negative thoughts and more muscle tension.

It's possible, however, to learn to recognize and to change your habitually negative thoughts using a three-step process described in Chapter 31. Similar treatments can be found in books like *Feeling Good* by David Burns and *Learned Optimism* by Martin Seligman, or you can get help from counselors trained in Cognitive Therapy.

6. Fighting Fatigue

Fatigue is the central symptom in CFS and a significant problem for most people with fibromyalgia. The term 'fatigue' may be a misleading way to refer to refer to the physical and mental exhaustion experienced by people with the two conditions. Manifesting as listlessness, sleepiness and a reduced tolerance for exercise, fatigue can be brought on by low levels of activity or for no apparent reason. Fatigue is often much greater than and lasts far longer than it would in a healthy person ("post-exertional malaise").

For people with CFS and/or FM, fatigue can have many causes. One is the conditions themselves, which leave people with less energy for daily activities. Other causes include:

Overexertion	Living "outside the energy envelope"
Pain	Ongoing discomfort leads to muscle tension, which is tiring
Poor Sleep	Sleep not restorative, compounding sense of tiredness
Inactivity	Less activity leads to deconditioning, so activity more tiring
Stress	Stress creates worry and muscle tension
Depression	Low spirits produce sense of listlessness
Poor Nutrition	Lack energy if don't eat well or have poor digestion
Medications	Side effects of drugs include fatigue

Here are seven ways to combat fatigue, matched to causes above. If you are bothered by fatigue, you can use the ideas below as a basis for your fatigue management plan.

Pacing

Perhaps the single most important key to controlling fatigue, and the other main symptoms of CFS and FM, is to adjust your activity level to fit your limits. This is often called "living within the energy envelope" or pacing. Rather than fighting the body and experiencing repeated cycles of push and crash, you seek to understand your body's requirements and to live within them. Pacing includes priority setting, rest breaks, short activity periods, switching between high and low intensity tasks and living by a schedule.

Each person's limits will be different, depending mainly on the severity of their illness. Dr. Paul Cheney summarizes this approach well when he says, "Proper limit-setting, which is always individualized, is the key to improvement." You can read much more on this topic in Part 3.

Another part of the challenge of adjustment is psychological: accepting that life has changed and learning to see your life in a new way. This acceptance is not resignation, but rather an acknowledgment of the need to live a different kind of life, one which honors the limits imposed by illness. In the words of one person in our program, "Getting well requires a shift from trying to override your body's signals to paying attention when your body tells you to stop or slow down." This process of accepting limits and learning to live a different kind of life usually takes several years and requires coming to terms with loss, the topic of Chapter 26.

Treat Pain and Poor Sleep

Fatigue is intensified by pain and poor sleep. Pain is inherently tiring and also tends to produce muscle tension, which in turn intensifies fatigue. Non-restorative sleep leaves you as tired in the morning as you were before going to bed. Treating pain and sleep using the strategies described in the two previous chapters produces the bonus of reducing fatigue at the same time.

The relationship between fatigue on the one hand, and pain and sleep on the other, works in the other direction as well. Treating fatigue can have a positive impact on sleep and pain. Since feeling tired increases the experience of pain, reducing fatigue lessens pain. In sum, fatigue, pain and sleep interact with one another. An improvement in one symptom can have a positive effect on the other two. Probably the most common symptom to attack first is sleep.

Exercise

If being ill reduces your activity level and leads to deconditioning, you may be able to start a spiral in the other direction with exercise. Exercise produces a higher level of fitness, thus reducing the fatigue caused by inactivity. It also helps combat pain, lessens stress and improves mood. For more, see Chapter 16.

Reduce Stress

You can combat the fatigue coming from stress by using relaxation and other stress management strategies, as outlined in Chapter 18. Because stress is so pervasive in chronic illness and because it intensifies symptoms such as pain and poor sleep as well as fatigue, many patients use a variety of strategies to combat it. Like other self-management strategies, stress management techniques improve multiple symptoms.

Address Depression and Other Emotions

Powerful emotions are part of chronic illness, a response to the disruption, losses and uncertainty it brings. Emotions can be treated using a combination of self-management strategies, professional help and medications. For more on this subject, see Chapter 19.

Improve Nutrition

CFS and fibromyalgia patients often experience several kinds of problems getting good nutrition. First, because of energy limitations, lack of appetite or severity of symptoms, some people may not spend enough time to prepare and eat balanced meals. Getting help, freezing meals ahead of time and using prepared foods can help.

Second, most people with CFS and FM experience an intolerance of alcohol and many are sensitive to caffeine and/or sweeteners. Cutting down or eliminating these substances may reduce symptoms and mood swings and also improve sleep.

Lastly, about one third of CFS patients, and a comparable portion of fibromyalgia patients, experience sensitivities to various foods or have difficulty absorbing nutrients. The most effective strategy for controlling food allergies is an elimination diet, in which foods are taken out of the diet and then reintroduced one by one as tolerated. For more ideas on nutrition, see Chapter 17.

Consider Medication Changes

Many medications, including some anti-depressants and drugs prescribed for pain, create fatigue as a side effect. A change of medication or a change in dosage may help.

7. *Treating Cognitive Problems*

Most people with CFS and many people with fibromyalgia experience cognitive problems, often called "brain fog" or "fibro fog." The problems include being forgetful, feeling confused, difficulty concentrating and the inability to speak clearly. Cognitive problems have a variety of causes, including:

Overexertion	Being too active, living "outside energy envelope"
Fatigue	Hard to be alert when tired
Poor Sleep	Fogginess created by not getting restorative sleep
Over-stimulation	Too much sensory information or info from multiple sources
Multi-tasking	Doing more than one task at the same time
Stress	Stress increases CFS/FM symptoms generally
Medications	Side effects include confusion and grogginess

Like the other symptoms discussed in this section, brain fog is best addressed by using a combination of strategies and by developing new habits. The strategies below are focused on combating cognitive problems, but your efforts to control other symptoms will also help you control fog. For example, because the problems associated with fog are found in people who are tired and those who are sleep-deprived, reducing fatigue and getting restorative sleep will help reduce cognitive problems.

Treatments

Cognitive problems are sometimes treated with stimulants, such as Provigil (modafinil), but these medications can produce a push/crash cycle. Here are 13 non-drug strategies for lifting the fog.

1. **Take a Rest Break.** Cognitive difficulties can be caused by overactivity. As one person in our program said, "Brain fog helps me to recognize when I'm outside my energy envelope and need a break." A brief rest may be enough to end the fog for some people. For more on the power of rest, see the article "Nurture Yourself with Pre-Emptive Rest" on our website: *www.cfidsselfhelp.org*.

2. **Avoid Over Stimulation.** If you are sensitive to noise, to light or to sensory input coming from more than one source at the same time (for example, trying to have a discussion with the TV on), limit sensory input by turning off the TV while talking, moving to a quiet place and avoiding distractions.

3. **Do One Thing at a Time (Avoid Multi-Tasking).** Many people with CFS and FM experience fog when they try to do more than one thing at a time, such as reading while watching TV or talking on the phone while fixing dinner. The solution: instead of multi-tasking, do only one thing at a time. To avoid interruptions, teach family members to wait by saying things like "I'm [fixing dinner, on the phone, etc.] right now, but I'll help you as soon as I'm done."

4. **Control Stress.** Stress can trigger or intensify brain fog. You can reduce fog by avoiding stressful situations, by learning how to relax in response to stress and by training yourself to mute the production of adrenaline. For more, see the chapter on controlling stress or the articles in the stress management archive of our website.

5. **Do a Medication Check.** Confusion can be a side effect of some medications. If you think this might apply to you, check with your doctor about adjusting the dosage levels of your drugs or changing to other medications. Also, discuss with your doctor the use of medications to increase attention and concentration.

6. **Use Lists and Other Reminders.** Write out your tasks for the day on a To Do list. Use Post-It notes in prominent places to jog your memory. Organize your house and possessions so that they give you built-in reminders. For example, keep your medicines where you dress, so you will see them and remember to take them when getting up in the morning and getting ready for bed at night.

7. **Organize and De-Clutter.** If you find your physical environment overwhelming, organize your house and remove clutter. For how to ideas, see the article "Illness and Housekeeping."

8. **Use Routine.** Reduce confusion by living a predictable life with routines: doing the same things every day in the same way. For example, always put your keys in your purse when you arrive home. If your fog is thickest in the morning, put out your clothes the night before.

9. Pick Your Best Time of Day. Do the tasks that require concentration and mental clarity during the hours you are sharpest. The best time of day varies from person to person. For many CFS patients, that time is mid-afternoon to early evening. Many fibromyalgia patients find mornings the best. Find the time that's best for you.

10. Postpone, Switch Tasks or Cancel Activities. If you're not thinking clearly, postpone jobs that are mentally challenging, switch to a simpler task or take a break. As one person in our program said, "When I'm too tired and foggy to think, I put things off until the next day and get extra rest instead."

11. Do Something Physical. Physical activity can increase energy and clear your mind. Activity includes exercise and other things such as laughing, singing and deep breathing. For some people, fog may be triggered by lack of nutrition. For them, eating counteracts mental fuzziness.

12. Reframe. Brain fog can be frightening and embarrassing. Many students have told us that they have learned to speak reassuringly or lightheartedly to themselves and to others at times when they lack mental clarity. If thinking you have to do something leaves you flustered, try slowing down. For more on reframing, see Chapter 31.

13. Plan Your Response. Deal with the fact that brain fog is confusing by planning your response ahead of time. Develop rules to guide you when you're feeling lost, so you have standard, habitual responses you can fall back on. For example, you might decide to respond to fog by lying down or by switching to a less demanding task.

Using Multiple Strategies

Like the other symptoms discussed in this section, brain fog is best addressed by using a combination of strategies and by developing new habits. When we have asked people in our groups to describe what they do to combat cognitive problems, we get lists that can be ten items or longer. Here is one person's description of how she handles cognitive problems.

> *My brain fog is worst when I'm exhausted, so I try and stay within my energy envelope. The fog episodes have greatly diminished since I learned that.*
>
> *Over the last several months, I've gotten organized. Orderliness helps to prevent panic and fog. And when I'm too tired and foggy to think, I put things off until the next day and get extra rest instead.*

I use self-talk too, saying "this too shall pass" or "nothing catastrophic will happen if I don't do this right now." That keeps me from going into panic mode and meltdown.

I'm mentally sharpest in the morning before I get really tired, so I schedule all my brain-heavy activities in the morning and leave the simple tasks for afternoon. I also nibble some protein every couple of hours.

PART 3

Manage Activity

8. Finding Limits: The Energy Envelope

Many people with CFS and fibromyalgia feel caught in repeated cycles of push and crash. Their symptoms and their reactions to them interact to keep them caught in a frustrating loop. (See diagram.) When their symptoms are low, they *push* to get as much done as they can and they overdo. But doing too much intensifies their symptoms and so they *crash*. The high level of symptoms leads them to rest in order to reduce discomfort. This is usually successful, since rest reduces their pain, fatigue and other symptoms.

But then, feeling frustrated at all they didn't do while resting, they plunge into another round of overactivity to catch up. This, in turn, causes another intensification of symptoms, so they experience another crash.

Living in response to symptoms, they are caught on a demoralizing roller coaster in which high symptoms alternate with periods of extended rest, and they feel out of control. This cycle can be especially frustrating for people with CFS because they often find that even small amounts of activity trigger a disproportionate increase in symptoms.

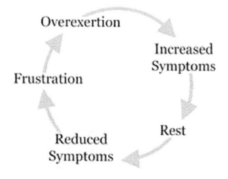

The Push/Crash Cycle

There is an alternative to repeated cycles of push and crash: pacing. Pacing involves understanding your limits and adapting to them. Pacing offers the possibility of a more stable and predictable life. With pacing, you can live your life according to a plan, rather than in response to symptoms, giving you a sense of managing the illness, rather than the illness controlling you.

This chapter describes the first of two steps to getting off the roller coaster: finding your limits. The next several chapters show you practical strategies for adjusting successfully to those limits.

Five Ways to Think About Limits

You can think of limits and living within them using a variety of images, metaphors and ideas. Here are five that people with CFS and FM have found useful.

The Energy Envelope

Imagine your life as composed of three elements. One is your *available energy*, the energy you have to accomplish things. This is your energy envelope. It is limited and is replenished by rest and food. Your illness has reduced it, typically by at least half. The second element is your *expended energy,* the energy you lose through physical, mental and emotional exertion. This is the resource you have to accomplish things. The third is your *symptoms*: fatigue, poor sleep, pain, brain fog, and so on.

In this view, if you expend more energy than you have available, you will intensify your symptoms. This is called *living outside the energy envelope*. This approach commonly leads to the cycle of push and crash. Pacing, which offers an alternative, means to learn how to live inside the energy envelope by keeping your expended energy within the limits of your available energy. Of the five ideas, this one is our favorite.

The Fifty Percent Solution

A second way to think about, and live within, limits is called the Fifty Percent Solution, described by William Collinge in his book *Recovering from Chronic Fatigue Syndrome*. He suggests you estimate how much you think you can accomplish each day, then divide that in two and aim to do the lesser amount. Rather than challenging your limits, you keep your activity to a safe level. The unexpended energy is a gift of healing that you give your body. Collinge's idea is a clever way of addressing our tendency to overestimate what we can accomplish. Another benefit is that it gives you permission to take care of yourself.

The Energy Bank Account

A third way to think about limits is to imagine your energy as money stored in a bank account. Because of your CFS or FM, your account has a very low balance. While healthy people are able to store up energy for a day's activity with seven to eight hours of rest at night, people with CFS or FM may get only a few hours of energy from a night's rest.

The small amount of energy available makes it easy to spend more energy than you have and overdraw your account. There is often a big service charge (intense symptoms) if you overdraw your account. Once you're overdrawn, you have to deposit more to your account in the form of rest. Alternatively, if you budget your time and control the amount of energy you spend, you can save some energy for healing. Vicki Lockwood explains how she uses this approach in her life in the article "My Energy Bank Account" at *www.cfidsselfhelp.org.*

The Bowl of Marbles

The bowl of marbles approach offers a similar idea with a different image. In this approach, you imagine your available energy as marbles in a bowl. Each marble represents a small amount of energy. You estimate your energy level each morning and put an appropriate number of marbles in the bowl. (Some people in our program have taken this idea literally, using marbles or coins stored in a bowl. Other people do calculations in their head.)

With every activity, you take one or more marbles out of the bowl: one for showering, one for dressing, etc. Some projects take more marbles than others. Also, the same task may require more marbles on bad days than on good days. Physical activity uses up your supply, but mental and emotional activity consume marbles as well. For example, if you feel frustrated about how few marbles you have, your frustration will use up some of your marbles. Stress, tension and fear are all big marble-users. Whatever you can do to lessen them will preserve your supply of marbles for other uses.

The Spoon Theory

Another way to think about limits, and to explain the idea of limits to others, is called the Spoon Theory. It is described in an article by that title written by Christine Miserandino, a woman with Lupus. (The article is posted at *http://www.butyoudontlooksick.com/the_spoon_theory/.*) She describes how she once explained to a friend what it is like to have a serious illness using spoons to symbolize available energy. She gave the friend 12 spoons to symbolize her energy allotment for the day. With each task the friend imagined doing, Christine took away one or more spoons. The friend used half her spoons just getting ready to go to work. Her friend "was forced to make choices and think about things differently." Christine contrasts her life to the life of healthy people. "When other people can simply do things,…I have to make a plan…Once people understand the spoon theory, they seem to understand me better."

Finding Limits

There are a variety of tools you can use to understand your limits. You'll find three below. If you are satisfied for now to have a general idea about limits, you can skip on to the next several chapters, which describes strategies for gaining control by pacing. If you are looking for ways to understand your limits in detail, read on.

Charting Your Envelope

You can get an idea of whether your current activity level is appropriate by spending a few minutes a day for a week charting your limits using the Envelope Log. This simple form can help you understand the relationship between your limits, your activity level and your symptoms. (See the sample on the next page and the blank form at the end of the chapter.)

To use the form, rate yourself on a scale of 1 to 10 for three elements:

> a) Energy level (available energy)
> b) Activity level (expended energy)
> c) Symptom level

On this scale, 1 represents, respectively, no energy, no activity or no symptoms, and 10 represents the energy of a healthy person of your age, a high activity level or the worst symptoms imaginable.

You can fill this out once a day or more frequently. Using it three times a day can help you see variations in your energy level and symptom level. You might find, for example, that your energy improves and your symptoms decline as the day goes on or vice versa.

The sample shows the form filled out for three days. Mornings are difficult for this person. On Monday and Tuesday the "am" reading for symptom level was moderate to severe. The sample also shows the push and crash pattern. On the first two days, the person kept her activity level within the limits of her available energy. Her symptom level dropped as the day progressed. Feeling good on Wednesday morning, she tried to make up for the days spent resting by "catching up" (activity level of 5). The result of her overactivity was a severe level of symptoms, starting in the afternoon.

		Envelope Log			
		Energy Level	Activity Level	Symptom Level	Comments
MON	AM	3	2	6	Rest
	PM	3	3	4	
	EVE	4	2	3	
TUE	AM	3	2	5	Rest
	PM	4	3	3	
	EVE	4	2	3	
WED	AM	4	5	3	over-activity
	PM	5	7	7	
	EVE	3	2	7	

Scale: 1 = no energy, no activity or no symptoms 10 = energy of healthy person, high activity level or worst symptoms imaginable

Establishing Limits One Activity at a Time

Another technique for discovering activity limits is to establish your limits one activity at a time. You may know that you get tired if you spend too long fixing meals, for example, or after doing errands or housework, or after talking to people. But you may not know when "too much" arrives. A way to answer the question is to focus on one activity at a time, keeping a simple record of time spent and symptoms.

For example, you may believe you can stand in the kitchen for 10 minutes while fixing meals. To test this idea, note your starting and ending time while preparing food, and how you feel during and after. If you find you are worse, 10 minutes may be too much. If you feel OK, you may be able to extend the time.

If you feel worse, it's important to understand why. If you are feeling weak or lightheaded, you may have exceeded your limit for standing. In that case, you have learned something important that applies to many situations. If you are in pain, you may have exceeded your limit for repetitive motion or may have held a tool inappropriately.

Discovering Limits with Logging

A good strategy for determining your overall activity limits is to keep a health diary or log. Record keeping gives you a way to record what you do from day to day and to see the consequences. A log helps you recognize linkages between activity level and symptoms.

Keeping written records can help you in various ways. A simple diary can show you how many hours of activity and what types of activity you can do safely. It can help you determine whether the effects of your activity are delayed and whether there are cumulative effects over several days or a week. For example, record keeping helped me to recognize that I often experienced delayed effects from exercise. I would feel no increase in my symptoms during exercise if I walked more than usual, but I had a higher than normal level of symptoms later in the day or even the next day.

Seeing that the effects of exertion were delayed taught me that I could not trust my body to send a signal at the time I went over my limit. This recognition also motivated me to use logging to define how much exercise I could do safely, so I could avoid symptoms by stopping when I had reached my limit.

Records can help you determine the varying effects of different activities. Some people with CFS or FM, for example, have difficulty with exercise, while others become nauseous after a short time on the computer, and still others become ill if they drive more than short distances. Your limits may be more restrictive in some areas than in others. Also, your pattern of limits will be different from that of someone else with CFS or FM.

Self-observation can also help you become aware of the effects of mental and emotional events, as well as physical activities. Many people with CFS and fibromyalgia find themselves easily tired by activities that require concentration, like balancing a checkbook, reading or working on the computer. Emotional events, such as worry, anger, conflict with others and depression, can be especially tiring.

Record keeping can help you recognize subtle links as well. For example, some people with CFS and FM have observed a surprising connection between their activity level and sleep. They find that if they are too active during the day, they become hyper-alert ("wired") and can't fall asleep. This is the opposite of what might have been true before they became ill, when lots of activity produced fatigue and a good night's rest. Counterintuitive realizations like this often come to light only through detailed records.

Developing a Detailed Understanding

While it's useful to think of your limits in general and call that your "energy envelope," in fact you have many "envelopes," one for each part of your life. You can gain further control over your illness by defining your limit in each area. Such an understanding can give you a thorough knowledge about what you have to do to minimize symptoms and increase your chances for improvement. It can also highlight your areas of greatest vulnerability, and thus help you set priorities for change. You may discover, for example, that good sleep is crucial to controlling symptoms or that minimizing stress has a dramatic effect on how you feel.

Your limits will be different from those of other people with your illness. Also, your limits will probably be tighter in some areas and less restrictive in others. For example, when I had recovered back to about 75% of normal overall, my exercise ability was about 35% of what it had been before I became ill. Also, your cushion or margin of error may vary from one area to another. Some people find that even small mistakes in some areas of their lives bring on a severe, disproportionate intensification of symptoms. For example, if they stay up an hour later than usual, they are especially tired the next day.

One way to understand your unique set of limits is to fill out the Energy Envelope form, which you can do after answering the questions in the rest of this chapter. You will find a sample form and a blank form at the end of the chapter. Printable copies of the Envelope form and all our other forms and worksheets are available on our website: *www.cfidsselfhelp.org*. Go to the Library and click on Logs, Forms & Worksheets.

The Energy Envelope form has five major sections.

Illness

This factor refers primarily to the severity of your chronic illness or illnesses. The pattern and strength of your CFS and/or fibromyalgia symptoms determine your safe level of activity. To get a good initial idea of a safe activity level, place yourself on the Rating Scale in Chapter 2. As a reality check, you might ask someone who knows you well to rate you, too, and compare the two ratings. We have found that, on average, people with CFS and FM rate themselves five to ten points higher than other people rate them.

The illness factor also refers to the presence of other illnesses and to the interactions between your CFS or fibromyalgia and other illnesses. Having multiple medical problems complicates living with CFS or fibromyalgia. If you have other ongoing illnesses besides CFS and/or fibromyalgia, record them on the form, too. Also, short-term illnesses may interact with CFS and fibromyalgia. One common pattern is for CFS and FM symptoms to be intensified by other illnesses, although sometimes there is a delay, so that CFS or fibromyalgia symptoms flare up as the acute illness is waning.

Activity

This factor refers to how much you can do without making yourself more symptomatic. We will examine activity in three areas: physical, mental and social.

Physical activity means any activity involving physical exertion. It includes things like housework, shopping, standing, driving and exercise. To define your limits in this area, estimate how many hours a day in total you can spend in physical activity without intensifying your symptoms. Because the effects of exertion can be cumulative, you might ask yourself how many hours a day you could sustain over a week without worsening symptoms. Also, you can note whether some parts of the day are better than others. Some people find activity may be safe during "good" hours of the day, but produce symptoms at other times. Then, estimate how long you can do various specific activities such as housework, shopping, standing up, driving and exercise.

Mental activity means activities requiring concentration, like reading, working on the computer or balancing a checkbook. Three questions to ask in this area are: How many hours per day can I spend on mental activity? How long can I spend in a single session? And what is my best time of day for mental work? Some people, for example, find they can work at the computer for 15 minutes or half an hour without problem, but that they experience symptoms if they work longer. They may be more productive at some times of the day than at others. If these ideas are true for you, you may be able to avoid triggering brain fog or other symptoms if you have two or more brief sessions a day rather than one long one or if you work on the computer only certain times of the day.

Social activity refers to the amount of time you spend interacting with other people. I suggest you think of social activity in two forms: in person and other (phone and email). Questions to ask yourself about each type include: How much time with people is safe for me in a day? In a week? Is the amount of time dependent on the specific people involved and the situation? (You may tolerate only a short time with some people, but feel relaxed around others.) For in-person meetings, you might also ask yourself whether the setting makes a difference. Meeting in a public place or with a large group may be stressful, but meeting privately or with a small group may be OK.

Sleep and Rest

This factor refers to the quantity and quality of both sleep at night and rest during the day. To understand how you're doing in this area, ask questions like: How many hours of sleep do I need? What is the best time for me to go to bed and to get up? How refreshing is my sleep?

Daytime rest means lying down with eyes closed in a quiet environment. Questions in this area include: How many hours of daytime rest do I need? How many rest periods do I have? How refreshing are my rests?

Feelings & Moods

This factor refers to the emotions we feel, especially worry, depression, anger, and grief. Questions in this area include: What emotions are important in my life right now and how intense are they? This factor also refers to the sensitivity we have to emotionally charged events and people. Some situations may trigger stronger reactions in us now than when we were healthy. These reactions may intensify symptoms because emotionally charged events can trigger the release of adrenaline, which often worsens symptoms.

Stress & Physical Sensitivities

This category refers to the sources of stress in our lives. Three are crucial: finances, relationships, and physical sensitivities.

The financial situations of people with CFS and fibromyalgia vary enormously. Some find their financial situation to be similar to what it was before becoming ill. For them, money may not be a stressor. For others, however, financial pressures can be great, even overwhelming. Some may live alone with little income. Getting payments from disability insurance may be a long and stressful ordeal. Those who succeed often worry that their disability status will be taken away. Others feel forced to work when their bodies are asking for rest.

Chronic illness changes relationships, creating new obligations and also new strains and frustrations. Your family and friends may or may not understand you. Relationships can be great sources of support and help, sources of stress, or both.

Physical sensitivities include sensitivity to food and other substances, vulnerability to noise and light, and sensitivity to weather and the seasons. Questions in this area are: Do I have allergic reactions to food? Am I chemically sensitive? Am I sensitive to sensory overload: noises, light, or stimulation coming from several sources at the same time (for example, trying to have a conversation with music playing in the background)? Am I affected by the seasons or changes in the weather?

Summary, Vulnerabilities and Goals

The end of the Energy Envelope form consists of three sections that can help you pull together what you have learned and plan for the future. The first, titled Summary, gives you a space to summarize briefly how you are doing at present.

The second, Vulnerabilities, asks you to focus on the factors that make your symptoms worse and those that trigger relapses. When we do this exercise in class, we often get answers like doing too much, poor sleep, financial problems, stressful relationships, uncertainty about the future, food and chemical allergies, sensory overload, time with people, family responsibilities, travel, and other illnesses.

The third section, Goals, gives you a place to identify the areas you intend to work on in the near future.

References

Arthritis Foundation. *Your Personal Guide to Living Well with Fibromyalgia.* Marietta, Ga: Longstreet Press, 1997. Explains the bowl of marbles.

King, Caroline, Leonard Jason, and others. "Think Inside the Envelope," *CFIDS Chronicle* 10 (Fall, 1997): 10-14.

		Envelope Log			
		Energy Level	Activity Level	Symptom Level	Comments
MON	**AM**				
	PM				
	EVE				
TUE	**AM**				
	PM				
	EVE				
WED	**AM**				
	PM				
	EVE				
THR	**AM**				
	PM				
	EVE				
FRI	**AM**				
	PM				
	EVE				
SAT	**AM**				
	PM				
	EVE				
SUN	**AM**				
	PM				
	EVE				

Scale: 1 = no energy, no activity or no symptoms
10 = energy of healthy person, high activity level or worst symptoms imaginable

Sample Energy Envelope

Illness

CFS/FM Rating	25
Other Chronic	IBS, Back problems
Acute	Secondary illnesses make FMS symptoms worse

Activity

Hours/Day	Two to four hours
Good/Bad Times	Good: late afternoon and evening
Housework	15 minutes at a time
Shopping	Use 'golf cart' at grocery store
Standing	Feel weak & dizzy after 15 minutes
Driving	Usually 20 minutes
Exercise	None
Mental per day	About one hour
Mental per session	Fibro fog after 15-20 minutes
Social: in person	OK if one or two people, in quiet environment
Social: phone	OK for 20-30 minutes if lying down

Sleep & Rest

Nighttime Sleep	Nine hours but not refreshing
Daytime Rests	Two two-hour naps

Feelings & Moods

Emotions	Worried re future; frustrated at how little can do
Sensitivity	Much more easily upset now

Stressors

Finances	Money tight: disability doesn't replace my salary
People	Husband resents extra responsibilities, daughter upset; Parents not understanding
Sensitivities: Food/Noise/Weather	Noisy places, changes in weather

Summary	Moderate to severe pain and fatigue much of time. Function only a few hours a day.
Vulnerabilities	Biggest problems are poor sleep and overdoing
Goals	Discuss sleep problems with doctor. Talk to husband about relationship

Energy Envelope
Illness
CFS/FM Rating
Other Chronic
Acute
Activity
Hours/Day
Good/Bad Times
Housework
Shopping
Standing
Driving
Exercise
Mental per day
Mental per session
Social: in person
Social: phone
Sleep & Rest
Nighttime Sleep
Daytime Rests

| **Feelings & Moods** |
| Emotions |
| Sensitivity |
| **Stressors** |
| Finances |
| People |
| Sensitivities: Food/ Noise/Weather |
| **Summary** |
| |
| **Vulnerabilities** |
| |
| **Goals** |
| |

9. *Pacing Strategies*

You found your limits by placing yourself on the Rating Scale and using the techniques outlined in the last chapter. Your next challenge is to adapt yourself to them. This is a gradual process, usually taking a period of years and involving the use of multiple strategies. Here are ten techniques to consider. Through experimentation, you can find the combination that works for you.

Reduce Activity Level

The primary strategy for adjusting to limits is to reduce your overall activity level. You can think of this as a two-step process. In the first step, you determine how much pruning you will have to do. For example, you can list the activities you do in a typical week, making an estimate of the time each takes. You then add up the times and compare them with the limits you established by using the Rating Scale or the envelope exercise in the previous chapter. If items on your list take more time than your limits allow (for example, you would like to have six hours a day of activity, but your body allows four), you will have to make some adjustments in order to stay inside your energy envelope.

In step two, you reduce your activity level using some combination of delegating, simplifying and eliminating. *Delegating* means finding someone else to do a task that you used to do. For example, family members might share in meal preparation or grocery shopping, or a cleaning service could take over housecleaning. Sources of help include family and friends, hiring someone, or using community resources, such as religious groups or service clubs. *Simplifying* means continuing to do something, but in a less elaborate or complete way. For example, you might clean house less often or cook less complicated meals. Finally, you may decide to *eliminate* some activities or relationships. For example, you can bow out of volunteer work or put some friendships on hold.

Take Scheduled Rests

Taking planned rests every day can help you reduce your symptoms, gain stability and reduce your total rest time. In contrast to rest taken as a way to recover from intense symptoms (*recuperative rest*), scheduled or *pre-emptive rest* is a strategy for avoiding flare-ups and escaping the cycle of push and crash.

Pre-emptive rest means integrating rest breaks into your daily schedule. The length of the rest period, the number of rests and the way rest is done vary from person to person. Many people take one or two rests of 15 minutes to half an hour each. People with severe CFS or FM may benefit from taking many brief rests a day, for example a 10 to 15 minute rest every hour or two.

You will gain maximum benefit if you are consistent, making rest a part of your daily routine regardless of how you feel. It can be tempting to skip the rest when you are feeling good. At such times, it may be helpful to remind yourself that, by taking scheduled rests, you are avoiding symptoms, and more rest, in the future. Resting according to a fixed schedule, not just when you feel sick or tired, is part of a shift from living in response to symptoms to living a planned life.

Many people find resting most effective if they lie down with their eyes closed in a quiet place, but others listen to music and/or rest in an easy chair. When you begin using pre-emptive rests, you may find you are distracted by your thoughts. If that occurs, try using a relaxation technique, listening to a CD or possibly reading a book. By focusing your attention on something other than your thoughts, you will relax your mind, making it easier to rest.

Resting by lying down with eyes closed is one of the most popular strategies used by people in our program. The important thing is to take a break from normal activity and to create a quiet place. Here's what one person in our program said about her experience with rest after taking our course: "Watching TV, talking on the phone, or talking with my family...I learned that these things could actually be quite tiring, even if I was lying down. Resting with eyes closed is completely different and, I found, very helpful. Before the course, I only *thought* I was resting; now I know that [for me] rest means lying down with my eyes closed (without television or the telephone)."

Scheduled rest is a popular energy management strategy because it is straightforward and brings immediate benefits: greater stability, reduced symptoms and greater stamina. A woman taking our self-help course told her group, "I decided to incorporate two scheduled rests into my day and the results have been incredible. My symptoms and pain have decreased and I feel more 'in control'. My sleep has been more refreshing and even my mood has improved." Another person said, "I have been resting in between activities, sometimes only for five minutes. For the first time in the four and a half years that I have been ill, I feel that it is possible to manage my symptoms and have some predictability in my life."

As noted above, some people find it helpful to take several daily pre-emptive rests every day, rather than one or two. One person who tried this was a woman with severe CFS who became tired with almost any exertion. It was as if her batteries ran down very quickly and needed frequent recharging. She was able to reduce her total rest time dramatically by using frequent short rest periods.

Before taking our course, she spent six hours a day resting, two naps of three hours each. After learning about pre-emptive rest, she decided to break up her day into one- and two-hour blocks, and to take a 10 to 15 minute rest during each block. Over a period of two months, she reduced her total rest time by an hour and a half. After six months, she had cut her rest time down to three hours a day. By resting in small blocks, she added three hours of activity time to her day without increasing her symptoms.

If you want to try pre-emptive rest, we suggest that you start with lying down in a quiet place. If that doesn't work for you, experiment with other ways of resting. If you fall asleep while resting, it may be a sign that your body requires more rest. You can determine your body's need for rest by keeping a sleep log.

Set Limits for Individual Activities

Another strategy is to set limits on particular activities. This can mean that you stop doing some things entirely or that you reduce the amount of time spent doing something so you stop before your symptoms intensify ("stop before you drop"). An example of the former is given in Eunice Beck's article, posted on our website (*www.cfidsselfhelp.org*), titled "Making a NOT TO DO List." Constructing a list of things you no longer want to do gives you permission to take things off your "should do" list, eliminating activities without feeling guilty about it. Having a "not to do" list gives you a justification for taking steps to protect your health. Eunice Beck includes in her list "not volunteering or being manipulated into commitments that I know will be a strain on my energy and pain level."

You can find an example of the power of setting limits on specific activities in Bobbie Brown's article on our site "25 Reasons Why I've Improved." The article describes how she increased her functional level from about 15% of normal to about 35% or 40%. Two items in Bobbie's list refer to medications, but most of her strategies involve changes in her daily habits and routines. She uses pacing techniques, such as taking regular, scheduled rests and living within limits. In fact, almost half her items are techniques for setting limits on herself, including limits on driving, time on the computer, time on the phone, sensory input, socializing, household responsibilities and travel.

To put limits on individual activities, follow a two-step approach. First, find your limits by experimenting using the technique described in the last chapter. Then gradually adjust your activities to fit within the limits. For example, you may set limits on how long you stand, how long or how far you drive, how long you spend on the computer or the phone, how long you spend socializing, how far from home you will travel, and how long you spend doing housework (or even which chores you will do). Some people find it helpful to enforce their limits using a timer.

Use Short Activity Periods

In addition to controlling symptoms through limiting your overall activity level, you can affect your symptoms by adjusting *how* you are active. Two short periods of work with a break in between can produce more and leave you feeling less symptomatic than the same amount of time expended in one block. Take a task like chopping vegetables. Some people may experience no pain if they stop after ten minutes, but pain that lasts one or two hours if they continue beyond that limit.

The same principle can be applied over longer periods of time. You may find, for example, that your overall symptom level is lower if you spread activities through the week, rather than trying to do many things in one or two days.

It is still possible to accomplish a lot even with very short activity periods, as shown by the experience of another person in our program. This woman, who is severely limited because of CFS, was asked to translate two documents. Through experimenting, she found she could work at her computer for only 15 minutes at a time before feeling ill. She decided to have four work periods a day of 15 minutes each for a total of one hour. She completed her translations in five months. Later, she was able to expand her work periods from four to eight a day.

Use Activity Shifting

Another strategy for getting more done is to shift from one type of activity to another, for example switching between physical, mental and social activities. If you find yourself tired after working on the computer, you might stop and call a friend, or go to the kitchen and prepare dinner.

Another way to use task switching is to divide your activities into different categories of difficulty, and to switch frequently among different types and schedule only a few of the most taxing activities a day. Here's what one person does: "I divide activities into light, moderate and heavy, and then plan my day to alternate activities in the different categories. By pacing myself in this way, I can do more and minimize my symptoms. In fact, I'm amazed at all I can now do in a day."

Use the Rule of Substitution (Pigs at a Trough)

It's easy to do "just one more thing," but this often leads to higher symptoms. The solution: think of substitution rather than addition. In order to add a new item to your schedule, drop one. For example, if your envelope allows you to leave the house three times a week and something new arises, find a way to postpone one of the usual outings in order to honor your "three times a week" limit. This approach is sometimes called "pigs at a trough." There is limited space beside a trough. The only way a new pig can get in is to squeeze another pig out.

Pay Attention to Time of Day

Most people with CFS and FM find they have better and worse times of the day. For some, mornings are good, while others perk up later in the day. It's likely you can get more done, without intensifying your symptoms, by changing *when* you do things, using your best hours for the most important or most demanding tasks.

Probably the most common pattern is a gradual improvement as the day wears on, with a slowing down in the evening. But, for some patients, mornings are the best times of day; for others, evenings. What is important is that you find *your* best time of day. One person in our program wrote about exercise, "If I walk in the evening, I can make it around two blocks, but three has me collapsing. Early in the day, I can do three or more. I have a window between 8 and 11 in the morning that is best for most activity, both mental and physical."

Another student was bothered by the effects of brain fog on her ability to read and retain information. Studying in the morning, she was able to read for only a half hour a day and had trouble remembering what she read. But she decided to experiment with studying in the afternoon. She found that she had good mental stamina for several hours if she started the afternoon with a brief rest. After her rest, she could read for two 30-minute sessions with a short break in the middle and retain the information. Over time, she expanded her study time to a total of two hours a day. Experimenting with time of day enabled her to increase her study time greatly while also increasing her comprehension.

Control Sensory Input

Many people with CFS and FM have an increased sensitivity to sensory information, especially light and sound. They find their concentration is affected by having too much sensory input. If this is true for you, you may be able to get more done and experience a lower symptom level if you focus on one thing and simplify your environment. For example, you may be able to understand what you read better if you turn off the TV while reading or move to a quiet place. If noisy restaurants bother you, try visiting during non-busy times. If you find large groups difficult, try getting together with only a few people. If media bother you, limit your exposure or have a "media fast," in which you refrain from watching TV or listening to the radio.

Sit When Possible & Use Devices

If you tire or feel faint while standing, consider sitting down whenever possible, for example to prepare meals and while showering (use a plastic stool or chair for the latter). You may be able to get more done, avoid symptoms or both by using devices to help you.

Some people with CFS and FM, who can't stand for long, who are sensitive to sensory input or both find shopping easier if they use a scooter or motorized cart. Many large stores have such devices, which they make available for free. One person in our program reported dramatic results from using a motorized cart in the supermarket. Prior to using the cart, she would be so tired from her weekly grocery shopping that she would lie down for two hours as soon as she returned from the store. If she shopped with the cart, she didn't need any rest at all after shopping.

Keep Pleasure in Life

Living with a chronic condition means ongoing discomfort and frustration. Pleasurable activities reduce frustration and stress, distract you from your symptoms and give you things to look forward to. Examples include taking a bath, having a conversation with a friend, listening to or playing music, seeing a movie, spending time in nature and reading. All can be considered pacing strategies because having enjoyable experiences makes it easier to accept and live within limits.

A Note on Accepting Your Limits

Pacing means adopting new habits, but it also requires making mental adjustments rooted in an acceptance that life has changed. This acknowledgment leads to a different relationship to the body, described by one person in our program as "a shift from trying to override your body's signals to paying attention when your body tells you to stop or slow down."

One part of this shift is changing our internal dialogue (self-talk) and expectations, so that they support our efforts to live well with illness rather than generating guilt. For example, one person in our program says that she used to think she was lazy when she took a nap. Now, when she rests she tells herself, "I am helping myself to be healthy. I am saving energy to spend time with my husband or to baby sit my grandchildren." Another person says, "I now accept the fact that I have a chronic illness and that this condition has, and will continue to, put great constraints on how I live. I now have a 'half life' but I am going to make it the best 'half life' that I can."

10. The Pacing Lifestyle

Pacing often begins with putting limits on individual activities or taking scheduled rests, but over time it can become a lifestyle as you learn to live according to a plan rather than in response to symptoms. The goal is to move gradually toward consistency in both activity and rest, doing a similar amount of activity each day and also taking similar amounts of rest. Implementing this approach involves planning in advance what you are going to do for a day and a week. To the extent you can live according to your plans, you will achieve a more predictable life, gain an increased sense of control over your illness, and may be able to expand your energy envelope.

Daily Plans

A good place to start is by planning a day at a time. In the morning or the night before, list possible activities for the day. Then evaluate your list, asking whether you will be able to do everything on it without intensifying your symptoms. If not, identify items that can be postponed, delegated or eliminated. One person in our program described her planning as follows: "Every evening I list my appointments and possible other activities for the following day. By doing this, I can recognize activities that I really don't have to do, but that can be postponed. This frees up my days for my targeted rest time."

As she mentions, rest breaks are an integral part of pacing. They should be integrated into your day as a regular part of your schedule. You will smooth out your life if you make rest consistent, setting aside certain times of day for rests of certain lengths of time. The idea is to rest by plan, rather than in response to symptoms

When you plan your day and live your plan, your symptoms are likely to come under better control and you may be tempted to do more. This temptation is part of the push and crash cycle that you are trying to break. Remember that the goal is to have a consistent level of activity, rather than to push hard when feeling well, then crash when symptoms intensify.

Developing routines is one way to increase consistency. Doing things in a regular and customary way reduces energy expenditure, because you are living by habit rather than continuously confronting new situations. Living your life in a predictable way can help reduce relapses, because routine is less stressful than novelty and because it increases your chances for living within your limits.

Your ability to do this depends on your developing a detailed understanding of your limits and then creating a schedule of activity and rest that honors those limits. One person who took our course said, "Developing a routine and sticking to it have been helpful because the familiarity reduces the number of surprises and lowers the attention that I have to spend on unexpected happenings. If I always wash my face after brushing my teeth, then, when I'm done brushing my teeth, I don't have to think about what I'm going to do next." For more on this topic, see the article "Habit Change & Rules: Two Keys to Improvement" at *www.cfidsselfhelp.org.*

Your ability to stay within your limits is complicated by the fact that your body may not give you a signal when you go outside your limits. You may feel fine even after going beyond your envelope, experiencing increased symptoms only later. Because the effects of overexertion are often delayed, you cannot rely on your body to tell you when to stop. The solution is to find your limits through experimentation and then limit your activity to a length of time your experiments have found to be safe.

The Daily Schedule Worksheet

The Daily Schedule worksheet gives you a way to translate your understanding of capabilities and limits into a daily routine of activities and rest. Adhering to the schedule offers a way to control symptoms and bring some stability to your life. (To get an idea of your limits, place yourself on the Rating Scale in Chapter 2, use the Activity Log from Chapter 30 or fill out the Energy Envelope form in Chapter 8. Any of those methods should give you a sense for how much activity your body can tolerate at the present time.)

Here's how one person made use of the Daily Schedule worksheet. Jane, who is married and in her 50's, contracted FM about 10 years ago and rated herself between 30 and 35 when she started our program, about average for people in our introductory course. She lives with her husband. Her two adult-age daughters live in the same city. Given her self-rating, she believed she could be active about three hours a day and could leave the house most days of the week. She wanted to work toward having a detailed schedule, but decided to start with just a few routines. Her initial priorities were good sleep, eating well and exercise.

Since getting good sleep was her highest priority, she began by writing out her bedtime routines. (See box.) The routines are aimed at helping her to relax before going to bed and also allow her to make plans for the next day, including her To Do. Having a list reduces her tendency to ruminate. Since morning is usually the time her fibro fog is strongest, she puts her clothes out the night before.

She decided that her morning and afternoon routines would focus on eating two healthy meals, stretching and taking pre-emptive rests. Since afternoon is her best time of day, she scheduled her daily outing then. (See the Weekly Schedule below for specifics.) The only thing she asked of herself during the evening was to prepare dinner for her husband and herself. (He gets his own breakfast and buys lunch at work.) The items she put on her schedule were not the only things she did during a day. Rather, they were those things she wanted to focus on at the time she started using the worksheet. As she succeeded with this first set, she added more items.

Bedtime Routines
Wind down: No TV, computer or phone
    calls after 9
Take bath
Make To Do list for tomorrow
Set out clothes for tomorrow
Take evening pills
In bed by 10

Morning Routines
Eat
Take morning meds
Shower & dress
Review & revise To Do list
Stretch
Rest for 20 minutes

Afternoon Routines
Eat
Stretch
Activity for the day (see Weekly
    Schedule)
Computer for 20 minutes
Rest for 20 minutes

Evening Routines
Fix dinner & eat

Weekly Plans

When you feel comfortable planning one day at a time, try moving on to planning longer periods, such as a week. The challenge here is to estimate what level of activity you can sustain over a period of time without worsening symptoms. Consistency in activity level brings control. You can find your sustainable activity level through experimentation. Maybe you can be active for two hours a day, four hours or even fourteen. The way to determine your limit is by trying different amounts of activity and noting the results.

I strongly recommend keeping written records. A health diary can reveal the connections between what you do and your symptoms. It also helps you hold yourself accountable for your actions, by showing you the effects of your decisions. And it can motivate you by showing you that staying inside your limits pays off in lower symptoms and a more stable life. For more on logging, see chapter 30.

Weekly Schedule Worksheet

Jane made use of a second planning worksheet: the Weekly Schedule. When she filled out the form below, she believed she could have one major activity each day without intensifying her symptoms. Since afternoon is her best time, she scheduled most of her activity for that time. She created the following worksheet as a typical week. She knew that if something unexpected came up, she would have to delete one of the items from her schedule.

Because exercise is important to her, she planned to go to the Y for a water exercise program two days a week. She set aside one afternoon for grocery shopping and other errands. Two other events were her weekly cooking, and time for laundry and housecleaning. Finally, she scheduled two afternoons a week for appointments or socializing. Her one evening event was having her daughters over for dinner on Sunday.

My Weekly Schedule						
Sunday	Monday	Tuesday	Wednesday	Thursday	Friday	Saturday
Morning						
Afternoon						
Weekly Cooking	Y Pool	Appts	Y Pool	Appts	Laundry Cleaning	Grocery Errands
Evening						
Family Time						

Jane soon concluded that her weekly schedule was unrealistic. She discovered that if she tried to do something every day, her symptoms were much higher and she had to spend at least one afternoon a week in bed. She decided to schedule two free days a week, with no trips outside the house. She also concluded that she could not both fix dinner and entertain her daughters on Sunday evening. Her body counted that as two events, which was beyond her limit of one per day.

Her experience led her to conclude that her true rating was probably between 25 and 30 on the CFS/FM Rating Scale, not the 30 to 35 she had believed previously. After thinking more about her limits and talking with her family, she came up with a revised schedule. (See below.) She switched her major weekly cooking from

Sunday to Saturday. At her request, her husband agreed to do the weekly grocery shopping. He and her daughters agreed to trade off preparing the family dinner on Sunday. Jane decided to free Friday afternoon for rest by spreading her laundry and housecleaning across the week rather than devoting Friday afternoon to them. She recognized that this experiment might not work and decided that her next step would be to ask her husband to help with chores or to hire someone.

Jane's experience is typical of people in our program. Adapting to CFS and FM usually involves experimentation and often tasks are transferred to others.

My Weekly Schedule						
Sunday	Monday	Tuesday	Wednesday	Thursday	Friday	Saturday
Morning						
Afternoon						
	Y Pool	Appts or rest	Y Pool	Appts	Rest	Weekly Cooking
Evening						
Family Time						

Daily Schedule

Morning Routines

_____   _____

_____   _____

_____   _____

Afternoon Routines

_____   _____

_____   _____

_____   _____

Evening Routines

_____   _____

_____   _____

_____   _____

Bedtime Routines

_____   _____

_____   _____

_____   _____

My Weekly Schedule

	Sunday	Monday	Tuesday	Wednesday	Thursday	Friday	Saturday
Morning							
Afternoon							
Evening							

11. Achieving Consistency

While most people with CFS and FM understand that staying within their energy envelope would bring a higher quality of life, many find it difficult to do. If you are in that situation, what can you do to increase your consistency in living within your limits? Here are nine strategies to consider.

Use Routine and Reminders

Having a regular daily schedule eliminates a lot of decision-making. One person in our program said, "Instead of having to ask whether something is or is not within my envelope, I have tried to stick to a schedule I know is safe." Another says, "Except in special circumstances, I do roughly the same stuff at roughly the same time of day….[I've done it for so long that] it's not a mental battle to do it - it's just the way my day is."

While pacing may seem daunting at first, it can become second nature over time as one's daily habits are altered. Bobbie Brown was able to do this, as she describes in an article on our website (*www.cfidsselfhelp.org*) titled "25 Reasons Why I've Improved." She first learned her limits for activities such as driving, time on the computer and phone, and socializing. Then she gradually altered her life to fit within the limits she had discovered. Habit change can be facilitated by using reminders. For example, you can use a timer to limit the length of computer sessions or post reminder notes on the refrigerator or bathroom mirror. For more on this topic, see Chapter 31.

Develop Personal Rules

Some people with CFS and FM have had success using detailed and individualized rules to protect them from doing too much. Living by a set of personal rules means not having to think and also reduces the power of spontaneity to overwhelm good judgment. If you are bothered by brain fog, you might consider taping rules in some prominent place, like the refrigerator, the bathroom mirror or your computer.

These may be general rules. For example, one person with a severe case of CFS has three rules for herself: no more than three trips outside the house per week, no driving beyond 12 miles from home, and no phone conversations longer than 20 minutes.

In addition, some people develop rules for specific circumstances. For example, they might set a limit on how long they stay on the computer, how long they spend with people in social situations and how long they will stand before taking a rest. If you develop specific rules for yourself, you can simplify your illness management program into asking yourself two questions: What situation am I in right now? What is my rule for this situation?

A related approach is, quoting the title of an article on our website, to develop a set of overall "Personal Guidelines for Managing Chronic Illness." The idea here is to have a few rules to guide your life with chronic illness, something you can turn to in times of confusion to guide you to a healthy decision.

Stop & Choose

One way that people get pulled outside their limits is by giving in to the temptation of doing something that seems appealing at the moment. A way to avoid such lapses is to stop before you act and realize you have a choice. One person in our program carries a card in her purse to remind her of the consequences of overactivity. On one side, it says "What's the Trade-Off?" The other side reads "Just Say No." (An alternative to the second part is to ask: "Am I willing to accept the consequences?")

Another person visualizes how she would feel if she went outside her envelope. She says, "Imagining the fatigue and brain fog provides a counterweight to the immediate pleasure I anticipate from doing something that takes me beyond my limit." A third person has sayings she uses to remind her of alternatives. One is "I can finish this task and crash or listen to my body and stop."

Alternatively, you can focus on the positive and give yourself reminders of what you gain through pacing. For example, you might post notes to yourself in prominent places in your house, saying things such as "Staying within limits gives me control," "Pacing reduces my symptoms," and "Pacing makes my life more stable."

Keep Records

Keeping a health log, which should take no more than a few minutes a day, can help you gain consistency in pacing in at least three ways.

First, records can help you get a clearer picture of your limits and reveal the connections between what you do and your symptoms. Using records, you can see how much activity you can do safely in a day and a week, and whether there are delayed effects. Also, a log can show the effects of mental and emotional events, as well as physical activity.

Second, a log can help you hold yourself accountable for your actions by documenting their effects. Reviewing your records can be like looking at yourself in a mirror. As one person in our program said, "Logging brings home to me the reality of my illness. Before logging, I didn't realize that most of my time is spent on or below about 35% functionality. This false perception that I was better than I am led me to overdo things, but now I am less ambitious."

Third, records can motivate you by showing you that staying inside your limits pays off in lower symptoms and a more stable life. Records of progress can provide hope. For more on record keeping, see Chapter 30.

Adjust Your Expectations

Many strategies for succeeding at pacing require the development of new habits and routines, which in turn are based on reduced expectations. The ability to develop new expectations is based on adopting a different attitude, a particular kind of acceptance. As explained by recovered CFS patient Dean Anderson, this acceptance is not resignation, but rather "an acceptance of the reality of the illness and of the need to lead a different kind of life, perhaps for the rest of my life."

Some people find it helpful to compare themselves to other people with CFS and FM rather than to healthy people. Coming to acceptance is a process that often takes several years, but it has significant benefits. In the words of one person, "I've discovered that I can now be perfectly at peace with lowering my expectations as I know too well what happens when I try to push the envelope and then relapse!!" For more on acceptance, see chapter 26.

Heed Your Body's Messages

You can gradually retrain yourself to respond differently to the signals sent by your body. Instead of ignoring your body, you can learn to hear and respond to the body's warning signs. In the words of one person, "Getting well requires a shift from trying to override your body's signals (in order to continue what you were doing) to paying attention when your body tells you to stop or slow down." Another person said, "I've had to learn to replace 'work until done' with 'stop when tired.'"

Make Changes Gradually

You may feel overwhelmed at times when you think of all the adjustments you have to make to live well with CFS or FM. The solution: focus on one thing at a time. One person described how she changed by saying, "The transformation into a more disciplined person was a long-term process. The changes have been introduced gradually over time. And I make sure I find the right one before I move on to adding the next."

Forgive Yourself

No one stays in their envelope all of the time. Life has its ups and downs; some times are more stressful than others. Instead of beating yourself up when you slip or circumstances overwhelm you, it's better just to ask, "What can I learn from this experience?" and move on. For step-by-step instructions for changing your "self-talk" (internal monologue of thoughts about yourself), see Chapter 31.

Value Yourself

Some people with CFS and FM have difficulty acting in their own interest. In some cases, the answer is to learn assertiveness. Assertiveness means finding your limits and then communicating them to others. One person in our program reported that she was able to avoid setbacks when she learned to speak up for herself. She wrote, "Communicating clearly when I need medicine, rest or quiet time and taking time for these things when I need them all help me to prevent a relapse." Asking for help rather than trying to do it all yourself is part of taking care of yourself.

Other people have a habit of putting others' needs ahead of their own. Sometimes called "people pleasers," these individuals with CFS and FM have difficulty setting limits or saying "no" to others. Because of this view, people pleasers may not take care of themselves. This trait can be deeply ingrained and may require counseling to change.

12. Travel and Other Special Events

Anything out of the ordinary --a vacation, a holiday celebration or even having people over for dinner-- creates a double challenge if you have CFS and/or FM. Non-routine events require more energy than normal daily life. For that reason, they can pull you outside your energy envelope, intensifying your symptoms. At the same time, you may want to be more active than usual or feel pressured by others to be more active, a second potential cause for a relapse.

How can you balance your desire to enjoy a special event with your body's limits? Here are four strategies, a success story and a planning tool.

Take Extra Rest: Before, During and After

Perhaps the most widely-used strategy for making special events more successful is to get more rest than usual before, during and after the event. Store up energy by taking extra rest before the event; limit symptoms by taking extra rest during; and take whatever extra rest is needed afterwards. The amount of extra rest will vary; twice as much as usual would be typical.

A member of one of our groups gave an example. If she is going on a one-week vacation, she plans for a two-week period. She makes sure that she doesn't take on any extra activities for a few days before and a few days after her trip. She also makes sure that she paces herself carefully during the trip, resting during her non-active times. After returning, she continues to take extra rest.

Another person reported a similar strategy: "It took me quite a while, but I finally realized the toll that travel and driving have on me. For a week or so before a trip, I double my normal daily rest time. I spend more than usual amounts of time resting while on vacation, and extend the practice for several days after returning. Also, I have had good success in reducing the effects of driving if I stop every two hours, tilt the seat back and snooze for 10 or 15 minutes."

Plan in Detail

Another strategy is to plan the special event in great detail. If you are traveling, this may include planning your activities for each day of the trip, including alternate activities you can do if your energy level is not what you expect. Depending on the severity of your condition, you might also arrange for a wheelchair or motorized cart in airports. If you are going to a family event, it might mean finding out the schedule ahead of time and deciding how much activity you will have.

One person in our program explains how planning has enabled her to stay within her limits while traveling. She says, "Making a commitment to myself to stay within a safe activity level has helped me resist the temptation to do too much when on the road. I can say to myself, 'I know you want to do this and people are pressuring you, but you decided before you came that this wouldn't fit into your envelope'."

Discuss Your Plans with Others

A third strategy is to talk about your limits to the other people involved in the event. After deciding on your level of participation, discuss your plans with the other people involved in the event, so they know what to expect from you. You might also alert them to the possibility that you may need to cancel out of some events and encourage them to do things without you at times when you need extra rest. If you discuss your limits and the unpredictability of symptoms with others ahead of time, you can reduce the chances disappointment and create a climate of flexibility.

Change Your Role

Another strategy for minimizing the cost of a special event is to change your role and level of involvement. One way to enjoy a trip or special event is by passing tasks on to others. For example, if you are accustomed to doing all the cooking for a holiday celebration, ask family members to each bring a dish. Or you might go to an event, but stay two hours, rather than the whole day or take periodic rest breaks. Travel can be made more doable by being less active than you used to be and by spending extra time resting.

These adjustments to activity are based on accepting a lower activity level and appreciating what you can do. As one person said, "I have benefited from the idea that half a loaf is better than nothing...Even if I haven't been able to do everything I did before becoming ill, making compromises has enabled me to participate at times somewhat outside my envelope so that I increased my symptoms somewhat but didn't suffer a bad flare-up."

A Special Event Success Story

A bedbound person in our program used several of these strategies to handle a ten-day visit from her daughter and seven year old granddaughter. This person, who has a severe case of CFS plus other medical conditions, was motivated to try something different because past visits had led to significant relapses. She prepared for the visit by reducing usual activities prior to the visit and using the time for extra rest. Also, she created a plan to alternate days of socializing with days of quiet rest, and explained her plan to her daughter, who accepted it. She spent time with her granddaughter every other day, but in a quiet way that did not overwhelm her. After her visitors left, she spent two days resting.

She looks back on the visit with a sense of triumph. Instead of repeating past experience, in which a visit led to a several-month relapse, the planned visit was an experience of control through pacing. About her time with her granddaughter, she wrote, "I had never even come close to surviving a visit from my granddaughter since developing CFS/FMS. It absolutely thrilled me that we were able to make some special memories together without it being damaging for me."

The Special Event Worksheet

As an aid to better non-routine events, here is the Special Event Worksheet. Use it to help you to plan how you will use your time during a special event and also the actions you can take in the period leading up to the event and the time after the event. The example shows how the worksheet might be filled out for a vacation.

Special Event Worksheet

Event: Family vacation

Actions Before:
Double normal daily rest time for one week before trip
No special events (e.g. nights out of house) for one week before trip
Decide on activity limits during trip (e.g. 4 hours per day)
Discuss limits with family

Actions During:
10-15 minutes rest every two hours while driving
Double normal daily rest time; take more rest if symptoms high
Maximum of 4 hours of activity per day

Actions After:
Double normal rest time for one week after returning home
No special events for one week

Special Event Worksheet

Event _____

Actions Before

_____

_____

_____

_____

Actions During

_____

_____

_____

_____

Actions After

_____

_____

_____

_____

13. Minimizing Relapses

Periods of intense symptoms, often called relapses, setbacks or flares, are a common and often demoralizing part of CFS and fibromyalgia. In addition to creating additional pain and discomfort, they can be deeply troubling, creating the worry that you will never gain control over your illness or make lasting improvement.

This chapter offers strategies to help you cope with the unevenness of your illness and its physical and psychological effects. You can apply the ideas to your life using the Relapse Worksheet, which is described at the end of the chapter.

Are You Having a Flare-Up Now?

If you are currently experiencing intense symptoms, ask yourself if your symptoms are familiar or if you are having new symptoms or symptoms with a new intensity. If your situation seems familiar, you may find the suggestions below helpful. But don't automatically assume that intense symptoms are just a flare up of CFS or fibromyalgia. A majority of people with CFS or fibromyalgia have one or more additional medical problems, and experience acute problems as well as long-term illnesses.

If current your situation feels new and different, you may have something else going on in addition to CFS or fibromyalgia. In that case, consider getting medical help. If your symptoms are very severe and acute, for example if you are experiencing chest pain or fainting, seek immediate medical help.

Limiting the Severity of Relapses

There are many things you can do to limit a relapse. Some are actions to take; others are mental adjustments to make the situation more understandable or bring consolation. Here are seven strategies to consider.

1. Identify and Respond to Warning Signs. You may be able to reduce the length of a setback, or even prevent it, by training yourself to spot relapse warning signs and to take quick action. Relapse warning signs are the signals your body sends that a setback is beginning. They include feeling especially weak, dizzy, tired or confused; having more pain than usual; feeling more confused than usual; and feeling cranky. Creating a list of your personal warning signs is one step in retraining yourself to pay attention to the signals a setback.

The second step is to develop a plan of what to do when warning signs appear, so that rather than ignoring your body's signals you can be responsive to them. Responses to warning signs may include lying down, reducing your activity level, limiting sensory input and/or limiting your time with other people.

A member of one of our groups said, "As soon as I begin to feel edgy, nauseous or tired or have muscle pain (all indicators that a relapse is imminent), I stop whatever I'm doing, go to my bedroom, draw the blinds and lie down. Then I practice deep breathing to clear my mind. This relaxation period can take from 45 minutes to over two hours. Usually, I arise refreshed and energetic, and can resume all normal activities."

Another person reported similar success in limiting the effects of migraine headaches. She taught herself to recognize the warning signs that a migraine was coming and, by making immediate use of relaxation techniques, she was able to decrease the intensity of the migraine or even prevent it.

2. Go to Bed …and Stay There. The most common strategy for overcoming setbacks is to take extra rest, continuing until the flare subsides. As one person in our program said, "When relapses occur, for whatever reason, I tell myself just to go with what my body is telling me to do: rest!" Another said, "One of my rules for living with CFS is: if all else fails, go to bed. This rule gives me permission to acknowledge that at times I am powerless over the illness and the smartest thing I can do is to give in to it."

3. Postpone, Delegate or Eliminate Tasks. Reducing activity by postponing tasks, asking for help or even letting go of something as unnecessary can help speed the end of a setback. One person commented, "Asking for help if I cannot do it all or just letting go of the less important things that I am unable to do at the time helps me reduce stress and my setbacks." Another commented, "On relapse occasions, I am not as hesitant as I once was to ask for help with either daily chores or whatever comes my way. I know my family wants to help me and it makes them feel good that they give me a hand."

4. Use Positive Self-Talk. People in our program say they are helped when they say consoling words to themselves during a setback. Because relapses can be deeply discouraging, it can help to say soothing words to yourself, such as "this flare will end, just like all the others." Self-reassurance can help you relax and quiet the inner voices that insist you'll never get better. For more on self-talk, see Chapter 31.

5. **Stay Connected.** Connecting with someone you trust via a phone call or email can be helpful because of the suggestions you receive, because of the reassurance you get or just from feeling connected to another person. One person in our program said, "It's much harder to be alone when I'm crashed, so I find a friendly voice on the phone for comfort." Another wrote, "I have found it very useful to talk with another person when I'm in the middle of a crash. Often it doesn't matter what we talk about; just feeling connected to something beyond myself helps lift my spirits."

6. **Prepare.** Having things handy and in place can help reduce the anxiety of a crash and make it easier to weather. Several people in our program have described how they plan for flare-ups. One keeps a large supply of food in the house, including food that her husband and children can cook. Also, she has rearranged her bedroom to have things she needs close to her bed.

7. **Take Extra Rest, Even If Flare Seems Over.** Long periods of rest can create frustration as you think about all the things you want to do, but can't because of your symptoms. This frustration can lead to resuming a normal activity level before the body is ready, leading, in turn, to another relapse. The final strategy for limiting the impact of relapses is to return gradually to a normal activity level. For many people, this means taking extra rest for several days after a relapse seems to be over. One person wrote, "When I feel the impulse to get back to work too soon, I visualize what I'll feel like if I do. That's usually good enough to convince me to take extra rest for another day or two."

Identifying Relapse Triggers

Some relapses are due to the waxing and waning of your illness, but other setbacks are triggered by actions you take, and events and situations that you can learn to manage or avoid. You can begin to gain control over relapses by identifying the factors that intensify your symptoms. To get you started, here are seven triggers often mentioned in our groups.

1. **Overactivity.** Living outside the energy envelope may be the most common cause of intense symptoms via the cycle of push and crash. The antidote: pacing. Living consistently within limits reduces the frequency and severity of relapses.

2. Poor Sleep. Non-restorative sleep can intensify symptoms and precipitate a vicious cycle in which symptoms and poor sleep reinforce one another. The solution: address sleep problems using good sleep habits, medications or both.

3. Travel and Other Special Events. Special events, like a vacation, a wedding, family visits or the holidays, can trigger a relapse. Events like these are often associated with expectations (both internal and from others) about our level of participation, leaving us feeling pressured toward a higher-than-usual activity level. But such events need not lead to a relapse. You may be able to minimize the cost of participation by making adjustments. For more on how to avoid setbacks by planning for special events, see the previous chapter.

4. Other Illnesses. Coming down with an acute illness or having multiple chronic illnesses can reduce energy and worsen symptoms. You can reduce flares by treating other conditions and acknowledging that they intensify symptoms. One person in our program said, "I've learned that I have to lower my expectations and level of activity when I have [an] extra illness, so as not to make this unavoidable relapse worse and last longer."

5. Stress. CFS and fibromyalgia are very stress-sensitive, so minimizing stress can prevent relapses. Stressors may include emotionally-charged events, such as financial problems, a disability review, a move or family conflict. Also, we may intensify setbacks by our expectations for ourselves or by our reactions to stress. For ideas on reducing stress, see chapter 18.

6. Stressful Relationships (Particular People). Some people with CFS and FM find interactions with particular people to be a source of disabling stress. Responses include talking with the person to redefine the relationship, limiting contact, getting professional help and ending the relation.

7. Sensory Overload. If you are sensitive to light, noise or crowds, you may experience intensified symptoms in situations of sensory overload. One common solution is avoidance. For example, get together with one or a few people rather than a large group or visit stores and restaurants when they are not busy.

Preventing Relapses

The last step in controlling flares is preventive: using lifestyle habits to avoid relapses. You can limit the frequency and severity of relapses using the eight approaches described in this section.

1. Pace Yourself. Pacing is a favorite strategy for bringing stability to life and preventing setbacks. The term covers a variety of strategies. At minimum, pacing means adjusting activity to the limits imposed by illness and to circumstances. As one person told us, "I've cut back my activity level substantially overall, and when I feel tired I cut it back even more."

Pacing may also involve having short activity periods. Particularly with tasks that involve repetitive motion, such as food preparation, you may avoid symptoms by breaking the task down into five or ten minute segments with a rest between each work period. The same principle applies to mental work as well, as suggested by one student who said, "I do stressful things like taxes in small bites. Letting them pile up just adds more stress."

You may be able to avoid an increase in symptoms by shifting among different activities and by including healthy activities in your day. As one person says, "What helps me is to have a balance of physical and mental activities, interspersed with frequent rests. I have recently introduced a checklist system to remind me about activities that are good for me such as walking, exercises, relaxing and hobbies."

Lastly, you may add stability to your life by living according to a realistic schedule. This involves both scheduling an appropriate number of activities and allowing plenty of time between activities, not pushing to squeeze in too much. One person in our program explained that she implemented scheduling by setting priorities for herself. She said, "It definitely helps me to make a list of weekly and daily activities so that I can prioritize them. I know how much physical activity I can handle in a day, so I remember this and make my list accordingly. I always allow at least an hour's rest in the afternoon so this is a given on my daily list."

Another pacing strategy is to have a daily routine. Living your life in a planned and predictable way can help reduce relapses for two reasons. First, routine is less stressful than novelty. And, second, having a predictable life increases your chances for living within your limits. Your ability to do this depends on your developing a detailed understanding of your limits and then creating a schedule of activity and rest that honors those limits.

Some people have had success using very detailed and individualized rules they created for themselves, as described earlier. A variant on this strategy is to write out a daily To Do list. Some people with severe brain fog find it useful to tape a set of instructions for themselves in some prominent place, like the refrigerator.

Another similar strategy is to have a series of rules for specific circumstances. For example, some people set a limit on how far they will drive, how long they stay on the computer and how long they spend with relatives. If you develop specific guidelines for yourself, you can simplify your illness management program into asking yourself two questions: "What situation am I in right now?" and "What is my rule for this situation?"

2. Rest. Scheduled rests, done on a regular basis, can prevent relapses. Also, taking extra rest before, during and after special events or after a secondary illness can help you avoid setbacks or limit their severity. One person in our program stated, "I can never get enough rest! The more I'm able to incorporate quality rest, even little bits and pieces, into my day, the better off I am." Another said about her use of rests, "I think my two daily fifteen-minute rests were the most important thing I did to aid my recovery."

If you know a time of unusual exertion is coming, something like a trip or a family gathering, you may be able to reduce its negative effects by taking more rest than usual for several days ahead of time, then having extra rest during the event and after as well. A woman in one of our groups adopted this approach to attend a wedding. For two days before the wedding, she had extra long naps and limited her activity. She arrived early at the wedding, having arranged ahead of time for a place she could nap after the ceremony. In the week after the wedding, she also took longer naps than usual and limited her activity.

Although she experienced some intensification of symptoms in the wake of the wedding, she did not crash. She called the experience a double success, since she both enjoyed the wedding and limited the price she paid.

3. Keep Records. Having a health log can reduce relapses in three ways. First, records help you define your energy envelope, giving you a detailed understanding of your limits. Logging can enable you to answer questions like: how many hours a day can I be active without intensifying my symptoms? How much sleep do I need? What are my relapse triggers?

Second, records can serve as a source of motivation. Seeing how living within the energy envelope reduces symptoms reinforces your successes and provides a motivation toward further improvement. Third, records can help you hold yourself accountable. Seeing evidence of a connection between overactivity and increased symptoms brings home the fact that activity level affects symptom level.

4. Make Mental Adjustments. Many of the coping techniques that help limit relapses require new habits and behaviors, but their foundation lies in new, lowered expectations for yourself that, in turn, are based on acceptance of limits. Here's what one person in our program said about mental adjustments she has made: "It has been important for me to accept my new life with CFS [and] move on. I've needed to redefine expectations of myself based on the new me. Lowering my standards and trying to break free from perfectionism has been a large part of this."

5. Honor the Body's Signals. There is a strong temptation to respond to the onset of symptoms by "pushing through." A different approach, listening to the body's signals, can prevent problems, as suggested by a person in our program, who said, "I have become more aware of the warning signals that my body sends me when I am doing too much and I am learning to stop as soon as symptoms appear - even if it's just lying down for a few minutes."

6. **Be Assertive.** Standing up for yourself can help you meet your needs, reduce stress and thereby prevent relapses. One person said, "Communicating clearly when I need medicine, rest, or quiet time and taking time for these things when I need them [all] help me to prevent a relapse." Another said, "It is extremely important for me to communicate my needs and limits to others."

7. **Embrace Solitude.** Time alone can reduce stress and allow for recharging of batteries. In the words of one person in our program, "Solitude helps me balance everything out. I have found it to be as necessary and fulfilling as resting. I get to know myself, tune into how I'm doing, and listen to what my body is telling me I need at that time."

8. **Control Stress and Pursue Pleasure.** Ongoing stress is one of the most challenging aspects of CFS and FM. You can control stress by using a daily stress reduction practice and other stress management strategies. Also, having pleasurable activities in your life reduces your frustration, making it easier to live within limits.

Relapse Worksheet

One way to gain some control over relapses is to use the Relapse Worksheet. It is divided into five sections. You will find a blank worksheet at the end of the chapter. A printable version is available online at our Logs, Forms and Worksheets page.

Limiting the Severity of Relapses

The first section asks you to state the strategies that help you limit the length and depth of setbacks. Here's an example.

> **Limiting Severity of Relapses**
> Respond to warning signs immediately
> Rest, rest, rest
> Postpone and delegate
> Speak reassuringly to myself
> Stay connected
> Have food in freezer
> Continue extra rest after feel better

Relapse Warning Signs

Relapse warning signs are the signals your body sends that indicate you are heading toward a relapse. If you respond by taking corrective actions (see the next section), you may be able to avoid a relapse entirely or at least reduce its severity. Having a list of warning signs can help you retrain yourself to respond differently when a downturn begins. The example to the right contains signals people in our program often list.

Relapse Warning Signs
Suddenly more tired than usual
Feel weak or dizzy
Extra pain
More confused than usual
Feeling stressed out
Cranky

Responding to Warning Signs

This part of the worksheet is your strategies for how to respond when warning signs appear. Having such a plan can help you to retrain yourself away from ignoring the signals of your body and in the direction of being responsive to its needs. Here's a list of possibilities.

Responses to Warning Signs
Stop: switch to less demanding task
Simplify: no multi-tasking
Lie down (get rest)
Get help with cooking, cleaning & laundry
Stretch
Go to bed earlier
Practice a relaxation procedure
Limit sensory input
Limit time with other people

Relapse Triggers

These are actions and events that consistently intensify your symptoms. Completing the relapse triggers form provides you with a list of your vulnerabilities. The example on right, which consists of items often mentioned by people in our groups, is offered as a starting point.

Relapse Triggers
Doing too much (outside energy envelope)
Poor sleep
Staying too long in one position
Travel
Secondary illnesses
Financial problems
Stressful relationships (particular people)
Worrying about the future
Light or sound (sensory overload)

Preventing Relapses

The last section focuses on prevention. It answers the question: what do I need to do to avoid relapses? The list on right contains ideas used by people in our program.

How to Avoid Relapses

Stick to my daily and weekly plans

Get to bed by 10

Stay within my activity limits

Limit phone calls to 20 minutes

Limit time on computer to 30 minutes per session

Limit travel to safe distances from home

Take regular rests each day

Exercise regularly

Take pain and sleep medications faithfully

Stick to "safe" foods

Ask others for help

Avoid certain people

Avoid noisy places (sensory overload)

Limit TV and other media

Schedule pleasurable activities

Practice relaxation and stress reduction every day

Relapse Worksheet

How I Limit Severity of Relapses

_____

_____

_____

_____

_____

My Relapse Triggers

_____

_____

_____

_____

_____

Relapse Warning Signs

_____

_____

_____

_____

How I Can Avoid Relapses

_____

_____

_____

_____

_____

Responses to Warning Signs

_____

_____

_____

_____

14. Pacing Success Stories

To give you an idea of what can be accomplished through pacing, here are two success stories from people with CFS: JoWynn Johns and Dean Anderson. JoWynn was severely restricted by her illness, but improved over a period of years by living within her energy envelope. Dean functioned at a higher level initially and eventually recovered. Both wrote articles about their experience that we have posted in the Success Stories archive on our website: *www.cfidsselfhelp.org*. For other pacing success stories, see the Energy Envelope & Pacing archive and the Success Stories on the site.

Learning to Control Symptoms

After a career as a corporate executive and management consultant, JoWynn Johns developed symptoms of CFS in 1991. In the first two years, she continued to live a busy life "despite feeling awful." From 1993 to 1997, a time she calls "all-out effort to get well," she experienced a collapse and responded by trying many different approaches, including exercise, yoga, meditation, homeopathy, special diets, medications and supplements. None of the strategies she tried helped her and she experienced repeated cycles of push and crash.

Two changes occurred during this period that pointed her in a more productive direction. First, she began to listen to her body, asking what it needed. Second, she changed her goal. Letting go of the idea of recovery, she focused on feeling better.

She began by asking herself what it would mean to have a good day. She decided that a good day meant having no minor symptoms and a minimal level of major symptoms. A good day also included being able to take a walk and do artwork. Because she found a strong connection between troubled sleep and bad days, she also developed a definition of a good night: sleeping at least seven hours and waking refreshed.

She then asked, "What do I have to do to have good days and good nights?" After studying her journal and notes, she concluded that she could have good days if she met six conditions: spending 12 hours a day in bed, getting seven hours of sleep, staying at home, restricting her daily activity, working on the computer no more than an hour at a time and having no visitors or long phone conversations. This was her energy envelope, her set of limits. (Her limits were quite restrictive, corresponding to a score below 20 on our Rating Scale. Your limits will depend on your unique situation.)

In the next period, JoWynn focused on developing a record keeping system. It included a monthly calendar, on which she noted her activities and symptoms, grading each day and night as good or bad. She used color coding so she could see at a glance how she was doing. Over time, she discovered patterns. Predictably, poor sleep was associated with bad days. But she also found that mental exertion and emotional stresses provoked symptoms just as much as physical activity. Explaining the motivation for her elaborate scheme, she said, "I needed to make this information visible to prove to myself the effects of mental and emotional exertion, as well as physical activity. I also wanted concrete evidence of the effects of staying inside my envelope."

She called the last phase "accepting my envelope." Living within her limits, JoWynn was able to greatly reduce her fatigue and other symptoms. Over time, she significantly increased the percentage of good days in each month from about 35% in 1996 to 80% and more in 1999. At the end of 2002, she wrote: "I now have nearly 100% symptom-free good days. What a difference that makes! For me, having CFS is like having diabetes: it's a chronic condition that can be managed and that requires lifestyle adaptations."

In 2006, she reported further improvements. She said, "I have adapted to CFS. It's been many years since I've been as sick as I was early on." She had not experienced IBS for two years and her sleep was noticeably better. Also, she reiterated her belief in the value of a self-management approach, saying "Over the years I've experimented with various treatments, remedies, regimens, supplements, and even, briefly and with bad results, some medications. None has made the slightest difference in my well-being. The *only* things that make me feel better and keep me relatively stabilized and able to achieve my priorities are scheduled resting and pacing."

A Recovery Story

Dean Anderson's approach was similar to JoWynn's, even though his starting and ending points were different. He functioned initially at a level corresponding to about 60 percent of normal and worked three-quarter time. After an eight year struggle, he returned to full-time work, travel and an active social life, and described himself as "substantially recovered."

Writing nine years after the onset of CFS, he reported that most of his recovery occurred after his fifth year of illness. He found that both attitude and actions were crucial to his improvement. To explain the former, he wrote that his approach to

CFS had changed over time. Initially, he believed that he could recover through determination and hard work, through trying to get well. Using this approach, he experienced some improvement, but he found himself devastated by relapses, which he viewed as signs of a failure of will power.

Over time, he came to believe that the key to his recovery was to adopt a different attitude, which he called a particular kind of acceptance. He described it not as resignation, but rather "an acceptance of the reality of the illness and of the need to lead a different kind of life, perhaps for the rest of my life." He explained that "the 'effort' required to recover from CFIDS is an exercise in discipline and hopefulness, not determination and striving." The required discipline requires a person "to recognize and adhere to one's known limitations and to follow a strict regimen without periodically lapsing….It is the will to protect oneself, to not over-do and to find ways to be productive and find fulfillment under unfamiliar and difficult circumstances."

He wrote that he enjoyed a good relationship with his physician, but experienced no benefit from visits with a chiropractor, a homeopathic doctor and an acupuncturist. He also tried various alternative treatments, but concluded that none of "the remedies, medicines or food supplements I tried helped me one bit." He came to believe that recovery would depend solely on his efforts and, with that belief, formulated a "recovery strategy." His approach included keeping a daily health journal, eliminating negative influences (both people and attitudes), and learning to be alone in silence (including learning to live without television).

A central element of his strategy was defining a safe level of work. Through experimentation, he found he could work six hours a day without intensifying his symptoms or jeopardizing his recovery. Although he continued to be quite symptomatic, he was successful in working at that level while improving gradually.

He sought out assignments away from the home office of his company, so that he could have better control over his daily schedule. He was successful in working at that level while improving very gradually. He used the hours freed up by his part-time schedule for self-care. He got out of the office for lunch and spent part of his lunch period resting. Also, he took an hour-long nap and did 20 minutes of visualization after he got home each day. He had other routines and limits as well. On business trips, he refused to take overnight flights, took naps after arriving at his destination and declined many dinner invitations. Summarizing his strategy, he said, "I gradually learned to pace myself to stay within my limits."

He also exercised on a regular basis, experimenting to find his limits in that part of his life, just as he had with work. He used a heart-rate monitor to assess the intensity of his workouts and kept records of "exercise duration and how I felt before, during and after each workout, and especially how I felt the next day." More importantly, he developed a new attitude toward exercise. A recovered "exercise junkie," he trained himself to enjoy exercise for its immediate benefits, without having any goal of progressing.

He also worked on his attitudes and emotions. He reports that during the first few years he was sick, he felt resentment and anger toward his ex-wife and others in his life, and also guilt and regret over past failures. His response was to work at changing his attitude so that he was not controlled by negative thoughts and emotions.

As he improved, he gradually expanded his work day and after eight years, reported "I have returned to a full and fulfilling life." He titled his recovery story "Acceptance, Discipline and Hope," saying he believes that what CFS patients need is the strength to accept their condition even if others refuse to, the discipline to do consistently the things that promote improvement, and an attitude of hope.

In Summary

Both JoWynn and Dean used similar strategies in responding to CFS. They both accepted the reality of their condition and the need to lead a different kind of life. They found their limits by listening to their bodies, by experimenting with different activity levels, and by keeping detailed records. Both had a flexible approach, in which they continually reflected on and learned from their experience. And they both found the key to improvement lay in disciplining themselves to live consistently within the limits of their illness. Their experiences demonstrate that people with CFS/FM may be able to exert significant influence on their symptoms and quality of life by the consistent use of pacing.

15. Job Options

Work issues can be among the most difficult to sort out. Should you stay in your current job despite the suffering or should you make some kind of change?

If you are on either end of the spectrum in terms of the severity of your illness, the answer may be obvious. Those who are minimally affected by CFS or fibromyalgia may be able to continue working full-time, accommodating to their illness by resting on weekends or reducing their social life. On the other end, some people are so severely ill that they cannot work at all. For them, pursuing private disability payments through their employer, government benefits or both may be the best course. (Disability is relatively common among people with CFS and FM. On average, about a third of people in our introductory course report they receive disability benefits.)

For those in between, here are four options to consider.

1. **Get Work Accommodations:** According to the Americans with Disabilities Act, employers are obligated to make "reasonable accommodations" for people with disabilities. Such accommodations may include making changes in work schedule (such as using flextime), getting ergonomically appropriate furniture or changing job responsibilities. Utilizing accommodations can be a way to test whether work is feasible. If you are unsuccessful in your efforts to shape your work to your limitations, you may want to consider applying for disability payments or some of the options below.

2. **Shift to Part-Time Work:** Some people with CFS and FM respond to their limitations by changing from full-time to part-time work. Working 15 or 30 hours a week is less taxing than having a full-time job, allowing for a less hectic pace of life and more time for rest. It may also allow for a more flexible schedule. Reductions in hours can also be accompanied by a changing to a position with less responsibility. Like reducing hours, changing positions can free energy for other purposes, although such a change requires some emotional, as well as financial, adjustments.

3. Take a Leave of Absence: Some companies allow employees to take a leave of absence for periods up to several months. Being off work can allow you to focus on healing and may help you clarify whether you can work and, if so, how much.

4. Change Careers: Lastly, you might consider changing careers to pursue work that is consistent with the limits imposed by your illness. People in our program have made changes to positions with less responsibility, to jobs that were less taxing emotionally and to work that was less physically demanding. Some have developed home-based businesses, especially ones that allowed them flexible schedules to accommodate the ups and downs of their illness.

One Person's Solution

Occupational therapist Kristin Scherger describes how she resolved her dilemmas about work in her article "Expanding My Envelope: How I Balanced Work and CFIDS." (Her article is posted in the Success Stories section of our website: *www.cfidsselfhelp.org*. CFIDS is another term for Chronic Fatigue Syndrome.)

After she became ill, her first attempt to combine work and CFS was to switch from full-time to half-time work, but she still experienced high symptoms and her life felt out of control. Next, she tried working as an on-call OT, but that was not successful either. "I would work myself to exhaustion, then require days of rest to recover. My life remained on a constant roller coaster." She felt frustrated at her patients. "The career I once loved had become a nightmare."

Over time, she recognized that she wasn't improving. Logging convinced her that she was outside her energy envelope. She rated herself about 30 on our scale on days she worked, but 45 when not working. She decided that if she didn't change careers, "I would never get off the roller coaster." She was able to achieve stability and expand her energy envelope by switching to an administrative position. She wrote about her new life: "My activity level and symptom level are now even better than those times a few years ago when I was not working at all." She rates herself at 60 most of the time and sometimes higher.

Kristin's story illustrates two themes we have seen often as people struggle with balancing illness and work. First, finding a long-term solution took some time. Kristin tried several arrangements before finding one that worked for her. Second, the eventual solution respected her limits. Her attempts failed until she found a situation her body could tolerate. Once the strain was removed, her body was able to heal enough to expand her limits.

Note on Disability in the US

Deciding when to apply for disability is complicated. Eligibility for disability is based on recent earnings, so waiting to apply can create a complication. If you switch to part-time work over an extended period of time before you apply for disability, you might lower how much you will receive under disability, since the amount of payment is based in part on earnings. If part-time work does not reduce your symptoms, it may be better to apply for disability quickly to maximize the size of your monthly benefit.

16. Exercise

Being ill reduces activity level and produces deconditioning, fatigue, pain, stiffness, anxiety and depression. One way to start a spiral in the other direction is with exercise. Exercise counteracts all these factors. It produces a higher level of fitness; it reduces fatigue, pain and stiffness; and it improves mood.

Exercise is usually an important part of a treatment plan for fibromyalgia and may be helpful for CFS patients as well. Before starting an exercise program, check with your doctor. He or she may refer you to other professionals who specialize in exercise, such as physical or occupational therapists.

A comprehensive fitness program includes three types of exercise:

- **Flexibility**: Stretching reduces pain and stiffness, and keeps joints and muscles flexible. Stretching is often a good starting place for an exercise routine and also can be used as a warm-up for other forms of exercise. Other types of flexibility exercises include yoga and Tai Chi.

- **Strength**: These exercises increase muscle strength, making it easier for you to do your daily activities. Strength exercises are often done using weights, but you can begin with simple movements like standing up from a chair or moving your arms.

- **Endurance**: Often called "aerobic exercise," endurance work strengthens your heart and lungs. This form of exercise helps lessen fatigue and pain by giving you more stamina; it also improves sleep and mood. Examples include walking, biking and water exercise.

Exercise: CFS vs. Fibromyalgia

The type and amount of exercise you do will differ depending on the severity of your illness and on whether you have CFS or fibromyalgia.

For most CFS patients, exercise can easily trigger an intensification of symptoms, so patients should focus on avoiding post-exertional fatigue (excessive tiredness after activity). All physical activity should be considered exercise. Even if you don't have a formal exercise program, you are exercising already (and may be overdoing it!) if you do things like clean house, wash laundry, cook, shop or garden. For more on how to identify what is too much activity, see box. Because many CFS patients have a tight limit on how much activity they can do without increasing symptoms, doing exercise might require that some other activities be dropped or rescheduled.

Exercise programs for CFS often focus on flexibility and strength; endurance exercise may be helpful, but only for higher-functioning patients. Pacing should be applied in exercise, so that a period of activity is alternated with rest. For some people, the time of exertion might be only a minute, followed by up to several minutes of rest.

If the biggest danger for CFS patients is post-exertional malaise, the danger for fibromyalgia patients is immobility. If you have fibromyalgia, fellow FM patient and author Stacie Bigelow suggests you think about a cement truck. The contents of the truck remain soft as long as they are continually moving. If the drum stops rotating, however, the cement hardens into concrete. She and other authorities on exercise for FM patients recommend two to five minutes of movement after 20 to 30 minutes of being sedentary. You can experiment to find what combination works for you.

Ms. Bigelow suggests that an exercise program for fibromyalgia begin with increasing daily activity, things like showering, making the bed, preparing meals, shopping, and taking care of children. Attention to daily activity should also include sensitivity to posture and movement, and to the pacing of activity. As noted in the chapter on treating pain, one way to control pain is through proper posture and body mechanics. Also, alternating periods of activity with rest breaks reduces the likelihood of exacerbating pain.

A formal exercise program for fibromyalgia can begin with stretching. Like being active, stretching increases flexibility, thereby reducing pain and stiffness. A stretching routine can be done most days of the week. (For sample flexibility exercises, see Chapter 4 in Bigelow's book *Fibromyalgia: Simple Relief through Movement* and Chapter 6 in *The Arthritis Foundation's Guide to Good Living with Fibromyalgia*.) A fibromyalgia exercise program normally also includes an endurance component, such as walking or pool exercise. You may use one or several types of exercise. Often, people with fibromyalgia can do endurance work most days of the week. Lastly, an exercise routine for FM should include strength

---

Heart Rate & Post-Exertional Malaise

If you have CFS, you are probably familiar with post-exertional malaise, the severe fatigue that results from doing too much. One trigger for malaise can be your heart rate. If it goes over a threshold, malaise will result. The threshold is often around 60% of maximum heart rate. (Maximum heart rate is 220 minus your age. For a person who is 50 years old, 60% of maximum heart rate is 102 beats per minute, calculated as: $[220 - 50] \times .60$.)

Some people can exceed their threshold easily with everyday activity. For example, one person in our program found that just going up a flight of stairs pushed her heart rate beyond her threshold. Another person says that lifting her daughter used to push her over the edge. The solution for the first person was to stop halfway up the stairs for a brief rest. The solution for the second was to sit down and have the child climb into her lap. A third person, who found that many activities put her over her limit, learned to be active with less exertion. She sits down for many activities in the kitchen, empties the dishwasher in stages, and uses a grabber to pick up things without having to bend over.

Staying within your heart rate threshold can lead to an expansion of the energy envelope. One person in our program reported, "I've made a lot of progress in the past year, mostly thanks to heart rate monitoring, which trained me to reduce my activity to a level my body can handle. By forcing myself to stay within my limits, I have slowly achieved an increase in what I am able to do."

If you think you might benefit from monitoring your heart rate, check with your doctor. For more on this subject, see the article "Pacing by Numbers: Using Your Heart Rate To Stay Inside the Energy Envelope at *www.cfidsselfhelp.org*."

---

training two or three times a week. (For sample strengthening exercises, see *The Arthritis Foundation's Guide to Good Living with Fibromyalgia* and Chapter 12 in *The Arthritis Helpbook*.)

Many fibromyalgia patients participate in water exercise classes. One example is the Arthritis Foundation's Aquatics Program, offered in many locations in the United States. For information, see the Foundation's website: *www.arthritis.org*.

Exercise Guidelines

In creating your exercise program, consider the following general guidelines.

1. **Individualize Your Program.** Exercise programs for CFS and fibromyalgia should be tailored to the unique situation of each person. The type, duration and intensity of exercise will depend on the severity of your illness and also will differ depending on whether you have CFS or FM. Your tolerance for exercise may vary depending on time of day, so it's important to understand how your limits are affected by when you work out.

2. **Set Realistic Goals.** Exercise has a different purpose for CFS and FM patients than for healthy people. Healthy people may train for an event like a marathon or work on sculpting their bodies. They can set goals and push themselves. That approach is likely to make symptoms worse for people with CFS and fibromyalgia. An appropriate exercise goal for CFS would be to improve fitness enough to make daily activities easier. For fibromyalgia, it is realistic to use exercise to reduce stiffness and pain.

3. **Start Low & Go Slow**. Begin by finding a safe level of exercise, one that does not intensify your symptoms. The goal is to have a sustainable level of effort that you can do several times a week. To improve your flexibility, you might try stretching, yoga or Tai Chi. For strength training, use light weights or isometric and isotonic exercises. (Isometric exercise involves tightening muscles without moving your joints. Isotonic exercise involves joint movement.) In the endurance category, many people with CFS and FM use walking and water exercise programs. For some people, starting low may mean as little as one or two minutes of exercise per session.

   It is usually advisable to keep the same duration goal for a considerable period of time and to increase the duration very gradually, as tolerated by the body. You may break down your total exercise times into a number of shorter sessions, aiming eventually for a total of something like a half an hour a day. It may take six months to a year to build up to a 30-minute routine; for some patients, 30 minutes is an unrealistic goal.

4. **Monitor Yourself.** The intensity of exercise for most patients should be in the 4 to 5 range, where 1 is resting and 10 is the most effort you can imagine. A standard often used to determine whether you have an appropriate level of aerobic exercise is the talk test: you should be able to carry on a conversation while exercising. If you have pain that lasts several hours after you finish, experiment with the intensity and length of your program. You may be able to reduce pain by experimenting with heat or massage before exercise and cold

after. Heat in the form of heat pads or warm water (a shower or bath) increases blood flow; cold in the form of ice packs or bags of frozen vegetables reduces inflammation.

To evaluate your program and troubleshoot problems, consider keeping a record of your exercise and the consequences. You might record the time and duration of exercise, its intensity and your symptom level before, during, after and the next day. You can note symptoms using a ten point scale or letters like L, M and H to note low, medium and high. A diary can help you see the effects of exercise, some of which may be delayed for hours or even a day.

Sticking with It: Exercise for the Long Haul

The benefits of exercise are greatest for those who exercise regularly. Here are some ideas for how to persevere with an exercise program.

1. **Do exercise you enjoy.** Your chances of sticking with an exercise program are much greater if you like what you are doing, so find a form of exercise you enjoy. Make your time more pleasant by listening to music or distracting yourself in some other way.

2. **Find the right setting**. If you have trouble motivating yourself to exercise alone, exercise with a friend or join a class. Making a commitment and socializing while you exercise are two good ways to increase the odds you will continue.

3. **Keep records.** Consider motivating yourself by keeping records. Setting goals and measuring progress often helps people stick with their program. Also, keeping an exercise diary is a way to hold yourself accountable.

17. Nutrition and Chemical Sensitivity

Finally in our discussion of activity, we turn to two other issues often encountered by people with CFS and fibromyalgia: getting adequate nutrition and experiencing chemical sensitivities.

Nutrition

People with CFS and fibromyalgia face several challenges to getting good nutrition. First, lack of energy, lack of appetite or severity of symptoms make it difficult for some people to spend enough time to prepare good meals. Some possible solutions include:

- **Being kind to your body in the kitchen**: Prepare meals in ways that respect your body's needs, such as taking rest breaks, using a stool, limiting repetitive motions, using good posture and avoiding dishes that take a long time to prepare.

- **Buying food online or by phone**: Replace visits to the grocery store with ordering from home and having groceries delivered.

- **Preparing meals ahead of time**: When feeling better, cook casseroles that will last for several days or freeze meals. Also, use frozen foods.

- **Getting help with food preparation**: Ask family members to share or take over responsibility for meal preparation or share food preparation with friends.

Second, most people with CFS and FM experience an intolerance of alcohol and many are sensitive to caffeine and other stimulants, sweeteners (such as sugar, corn syrup, fructose, aspartame and saccharin), food additives (such as MSG, preservatives, artificial colors and artificial flavors) and tobacco. Cutting down or eliminating these substances may reduce symptoms and mood swings, and also improve sleep.

Third, about one third of CFS and fibromyalgia patients experience food sensitivities or food allergies or have difficulty absorbing nutrients. Negative reactions include gastrointestinal symptoms (such as heartburn, gas, nausea, diarrhea and constipation), headaches, muscle pain, changes in pulse and fatigue.

Unfortunately, there is no common set of foods to which susceptible CFS and FM patients are sensitive. One person may respond badly to dairy, while another must avoid wheat. Some common sources of food allergy include dairy products, eggs, soy, wheat and corn. Other sources include tomatoes, potatoes and other members of the nightshade family; fruits; spicy foods; gas-producing vegetables, such as onions, cabbage and broccoli; raw foods; and nuts.

There are two major treatments for food sensitivities and allergies: avoidance and the rotation diet. The first step in both treatments is the same: identifying foods that trigger allergic reactions. To do this, list foods you think might cause problems, eliminate them from your diet, and then reintroduce them one by one. Because reactions can take one to several days to develop, you will need to record what foods you eat and what symptoms you experience for a several-day period.

If foods produce strong reactions, such as diarrhea, nausea, headaches or hives, you will probably have to eliminate them from your diet entirely. Often, the elimination of just a few foods can improve symptoms dramatically. Alternatively, you may find you can tolerate a food if you eat it only occasionally. After eating a food, you wait a period of four to seven days before eating it again.

As with so much concerning CFS and fibromyalgia, reactions to food are highly individual, so there is no off-the-shelf, standard "CFS diet" or "fibromyalgia diet." Here are five general guidelines.

1. **Experiment.** About two thirds of CFS and FM patients don't have food allergies and can focus on getting a balanced diet and avoiding substances such as alcohol and tobacco. The remainder will have to work to find the foods to which they are sensitive. Because reactions to food vary from person to person, people in this third have to experiment to determine the foods that create reactions and then experiment to determine whether to reduce or eliminate them from the diet.

2. **Listen to your body.** If a food or substance makes you feel worse, don't eat it. Sensitivities vary tremendously; it's possible that you might not tolerate "good foods" such as some fruits and vegetables.

3. **Eat sensibly.** To the extent allowed by your sensitivities, eat a balanced diet. There is more danger in trying fad diets than in eating a standard diet generally recommended for all adults, one that is moderate in fat and includes a variety of foods from different food groups, focusing on fruits, vegetables, whole grains.

4. Avoid some foods and substances. Almost all people with CFS and FM are intolerant of alcohol and stimulants like the caffeine found in coffee and tea. Many are sensitive to sweeteners and food additives. Eliminating or reducing these products makes sense for most people with the two conditions.

5. Consider other causes of food problems. Many CFS and FM patients also suffer from irritable bowel syndrome (IBS); yeast infections, like candida; celiac disease, which causes a strong allergic reaction to wheat and other grains; and lactose intolerance, which is the inability to digest the sugar in milk. Consider whether some or all of your food sensitivities might be caused by these other illnesses.

Chemical Sensitivities

A significant number of people with CFS and FM experience allergic reactions to other substances besides food. The range of reactions varies greatly among patients, from mild annoyance to serious threat. Those on the far end of the spectrum may be housebound because of their sensitivities.

Sensitivities to mold, dust mites and grasses are common. People also react to perfumes, scented products, cigarette smoke, household chemicals, car exhaust and diesel fumes, glues, inks and dyes. Symptoms include headaches, dizziness, faintness and nausea. (Because many patients are chemically sensitive, most CFS and FM support groups ask people to come "fragrance free.")

The most useful coping strategy is avoidance, which includes eliminating offending substances from the home and limiting exposure to them while outside the house. If you think you might be chemically sensitive, check the products in your kitchen, bathroom and laundry, such as cleaners, soaps, detergents, pesticides and personal care products, such as deodorants, shampoos, toothpaste, lotions and perfumes. For more, see Chapters 8 and 9 in Erica Verrillo and Lauren Gellman's book *Chronic Fatigue Syndrome: A Treatment Guide* and the discussion on designing a healthy environment in Fred Friedberg's book *Coping with Chronic Fatigue Syndrome*.

PART 4

Reduce Stress and Manage Feelings

18. Controlling Stress

Stress is a double challenge for people with Chronic Fatigue Syndrome and fibromyalgia. Illness adds new sources of stress, such as the ongoing discomfort of symptoms, uncertainty about the future and financial pressure. In addition, CFS and FM are very stress-sensitive illnesses, so that the effects of a given level of stress are greater than they would be for a healthy person.

Thus, you face a double challenge related to stress: your stresses are multiplied at a time when you are more vulnerable to the effects of stress. This combination makes addressing stress a high priority. By using stress management techniques such as those described in this chapter, you can learn how to interrupt the cycle in which symptoms and stress reinforce one another.

Sources and Signs of Stress

One reason that stress is such a big challenge in CFS and FM is that it can come from many different sources. They include:

Symptoms	Ongoing discomfort is debilitating and worrisome
Limits	Frustration due to smaller energy envelope
Loss	Many losses: health, income, friends, etc.
Isolation	Stress from time alone and from feeling different
Money	Financial pressure
Relationships	Often strained; some may end
Thoughts	Unrealistic expectations or feeling helpless
Uncertainty	Worry about the future
Sound & Light	Sensitivity to sense data
Allergies	Sensitivity to foods and/or chemicals

Any of the following can indicate that you are under stress.

- Muscle tension (especially in head, neck & shoulders)
- Feeling anxious or nervous
- Moodiness
- Feeling depressed
- Nervous movement (e.g. tapping fingers or feet)
- Irritability
- Sleep problems (trouble falling asleep or staying asleep)
- Grinding teeth or clenching jaw

Approaches to Managing Stress

Because stress is so common and so debilitating, we recommend that people with CFS and FM use multiple techniques to manage it. Many people in our program manage stress with pacing strategies such as reducing their activity level, learning to say "no," taking daily rests and using routine. Some describe a change in their employment situation as a stress reduction measure. These work changes have included switching from full-time to part-time work, moving to a less demanding job, working from home, adopting a flexible schedule, and taking early retirement.

Other frequently-used approaches include doing a daily relaxation procedure, de-cluttering (e.g. reorganizing the kitchen or discarding unused possessions), limiting exposure to the media, limiting contact with some people, avoiding crowds, getting help with household chores and making mental adjustments (such as letting go of unrealistic expectations).

Because there are so many causes of stress, it pays to use a variety of approaches to manage it. One person in our program says, "I do a variety of things to manage stress, such as deep breathing, listening to relaxation tapes, getting regular massages, walking with my dog, and writing in my journal." Another writes, "The ways I try to handle stress are: meditating daily, scheduling a regular time [to go to] bed each night, keeping our home an emotionally welcoming place for my husband, engaging in pleasurable activities, and avoiding unwanted situations [that] drain my energy."

We will explore two categories stress management: *stress reduction* and *stress avoidance*. The first involves retraining yourself, learning how to respond differently to stressors so that they do not have the same effect as in the past. The second approach is preventive, taking measures to avoid stressful circumstances.

Stress Reduction

Often, how we view and react to a stressor determines how much stress we experience. For example, if you worry in response to an increase in symptoms, you may tense your muscles. Muscle tension can create pain, draining energy and causing fatigue. By learning to relax, you can lessen muscle tension and ease symptoms. This is one example of how to reduce the impact of stressors by changing your response. Here are 14 stress reduction strategies to consider.

Relaxation

When we become stressed in the face of challenge, we often respond with a fight-or-flight reaction. Adrenaline flows, and we feel charged up. If the challenge is brief, the initial reaction is followed by relaxation. If, however, you feel yourself to be under constant threat, as you may if you are always in pain, your body stays in a state of tension.

Physically relaxing activities counteract both the physical and the emotional aspects of stress. Through relaxation, you can reduce muscle tension and anxiety. Relaxation is also very helpful for pain control. Combining rest with a relaxation procedure or meditation can be an even more effective means of stress reduction.

Examples of stress reduction procedures include focusing on your breathing, the body scan, progressive relaxation, and guided imagery. (You can find step-by-step instructions for these and other relaxation procedures in the predecessor to this book, available in the Online Books section of our website: *www.cfidsselfhelp.org*.) Because everyone is different, some techniques work well for one person and other techniques work better for another. In particular, techniques using imagery seem very helpful to some people, but not useful to others. Try several techniques to see what works for you. Also, you may find that a particular technique works for a while, and then becomes ineffective. If that happens, try something else.

It usually takes several weeks or more of practice to develop skill in using a technique, so allow some time before expecting results. To be fair, you should practice four or five times a week, setting aside ten to 20 minutes for each session and choosing a time when you won't be disturbed. Learning concentration is a common problem when doing a relaxation practice. The mind tends to wander, so having patience is necessary.

There are many good relaxation and meditation tapes available today. Some have step-by-step instructions to lead you through a relaxation procedure, while others have music or relaxing sounds from nature. You may want to use such tapes or record your own from the techniques you find on our website or elsewhere. If relaxation makes you anxious or seems unpleasant, try other stress reduction techniques.

Formal relaxation procedures work for many people, but other, less formal approaches can help, too. These include exercise, baths, massage, acupuncture, rest and listening to music.

Mental Adjustments

Your thoughts can be another source of stress. For example, you may have unrealistic expectations for yourself. You may think that, as a "good mother" or "good wife," you should keep the house as you did before becoming ill. If that's the case, you can reduce suffering by changing your expectations, so they better match your current abilities. A number of people in our program refer to themselves as "recovering perfectionists." Becoming aware of and changing the standards you have for yourself reduces stress and helps you avoid overdoing.

It may also help to change your expectations about how others view you. As one person said, "I let go of expecting people to respond to me the way I think they 'should'. For example, I let go of expecting that people will understand my disease. So with no expectations, I [feel] less resentment, which leads to less stress in life."

Thoughts can increase stress is through our "self-talk," the internal dialogue we have with ourselves, especially about negative events. For some people, an increase in symptoms may trigger thoughts like "I'm not getting anywhere," "I'll never get better" or "It's hopeless." Negative thoughts like these can then make you feel anxious, sad and helpless. The thoughts and the stress they create may make your symptoms worse and trigger another round of negative thoughts. The cycle can be very demoralizing, leading to an overly pessimistic view of your situation and making it difficult to motivate yourself to do things to feel better.

But you can learn how to recognize and change habitual negative thoughts so that your self-talk is more realistic and more positive. There are many self-help manuals for doing this. Our favorite is the one by Greenberger and Padesky. (See References, at the end of the chapter.) Others include books by Burns and Seligman. Also, you can get professional help; look for a counselor who specializes in Cognitive Therapy, also called Cognitive Behavioral Therapy (CBT). For an introduction to Cognitive Therapy, see Chapter 31.

Supportive Relationships: Family, Friends and Professionals

Good relations are a buffer against stress. Feeling connected to people who understand and respect you reduces anxiety and counteracts depression. Beyond that, talking to another person may help you clarify your situation or the response you receive may enable you to see your life in a different, more constructive way. You may receive such support from family members, friends, other people with CFS and FM or therapists. Support also means practical assistance, which might include such things as shopping, cooking, bill paying or housecleaning. For more on this topic, see the section on relationships.

Problem Solving

Taking practical steps to improve your situation can also help reduce anxiety and worry. A member of one of our groups, who suffers from severe brain fog, reported that she had gone to the emergency room after taking her medications three times in one day. Worried that brain fog might lead her to make the same mistake again, she asked her group for suggestions and adopted one of them: a pill box with compartments for each day of the week. She reported that the pillbox was a stress minimizer, greatly reducing her fear of repeating her mistake.

Another person in our program reported, "I have spent quite a bit of time analyzing my activities, everything from how long I stayed somewhere to ways to minimize pain in doing chores. From this analysis, I have tried many different ideas that have proved to be very helpful, such as a book holder for the newspaper."

Information

Educating yourself about CFS and FM can be a great stress reducer, as you replace fears with facts. Two places to start, on our website *www.cfidsselfhelp.org*, are the Basic Facts About CFS and FM link on the homepage and the article "Educate Yourself" which is part of the series "Eight Steps to a Better Life."

Pleasurable Activities

Doing things that bring you pleasure can distract you from stress and reduce preoccupation with problems. Listening to or playing music or engaging in other artistic pursuits are good stress reducers. The same can be said of reading a good book, seeing an engrossing movie, spending time in nature and talking with a friend. The key is to find an activity in which you can become absorbed. By immersing yourself, you interrupt the worry cycle, distract yourself from symptoms and experience some relaxing pleasure.

Exercise and Movement

Exercise is a natural stress reducer, since it causes your body to produce endorphins and other soothing body chemicals. A similar effect can be obtained through other forms of movement. If you are worried, just getting up and moving around can help break the spell.

Journaling

Writing may be useful as a stress reducer. You might find it helpful to write out what's bothering you as a way of venting frustration and lessening worry. Another use of journaling is to help you change perspective on your life. Some people have told us they found it very helpful to keep a journal in which they note positive events every day. Over time, they found that their mental attitude toward their illness and their life changed in a positive direction. See Joan Buchman's article "The Healing Power of Gratitude" on our website: *www.cfidsselfhelp.org.* For a model of a gratitude journal, see Sarah Ban Breathnach's book *Simple Abundance Journal of Gratitude*.

Talking and Being Listened To

It is not surprising that, in a survey, talking to a friend was rated as the number one way to combat worry. Talking to someone you trust provides reassurance and connectedness to dispel worry. According to Edward Hallowell, studies have shown that talking to another person changes what is happening in your brain at a physical level.

Laughter and Humor

This is another good stress reducer. Watching a funny movie, reading a humorous book, looking at favorite cartoons or laughing with friends can be a great release. Like exercise, laughter promotes the production of endorphins, brain chemicals that produce good feelings and reduce pain. Research suggests that it can strengthen the immune system, counteract depression and even provide a substitute for aerobic exercise. Short periods of laughter can double your heart rate for three to five minutes. A natural tension reducer, laughter produces relaxation for up to 45 minutes.

Solitude

For some people, just having time alone can be helpful. One person wrote, "I spend much of my time in quiet, relaxing activities such as reading, needlework, etc. If I have a day that does not allow me to participate in these activities to some minimal extent, I find myself extremely tense, stressed out and emotional."

Assertiveness

By speaking up for yourself, setting limits and saying "No," you protect yourself and avoid doing things that intensify symptoms. For example, you can teach your family and friends to respect your need for rest times and can make your limits clear by telling others how long you'll talk on the phone or how much time you will spend at a party. By having a "voice," you reduce the stress that results from keepings things inside.

Also, learn to delegate and ask for help. Others often feel as helpless as you about your illness; asking them to help you in some specific way replaces the sense of helplessness with a feeling of accomplishment.

Medications

Prescription medications can be helpful as part of a stress management program. As one person in our program wrote, "I resisted the idea [of medications] for a long time, and now kick myself for having done so. [Zoloft] has helped level off my reactions to everyday stress and evened out my mood."

Stress Avoidance

Stress avoidance is preventive, using self-observation to learn how stress affects you and then taking measures to avoid stressful circumstances. For example, you may notice that when you hit a limit, any further activity will intensify your symptoms. In such circumstances, rest can reduce the stress on your body. Having good relationships are a buffer against stress. People with supportive relationships have lower anxiety and depression.

Overall, the idea of prevention is to avoid generating a stress response by avoiding stressful situations. Fewer stress hormones means more time for your body to repair itself. The main ways that people in our groups prevent stress are by avoiding stress triggers and by using pacing, order and routine.

Avoiding Stress Triggers

There are three types of stress triggers: substances that create allergic reactions, situations that produce sensory overload and certain people. You can reduce symptoms by avoiding foods and other substances to which you are allergic or sensitive, minimizing situations that create sensory overload and limiting contact with anxious, negative or overly-demanding people.

If you are particularly sensitive to light, noise or crowds, or experience sensory overload in other ways, avoiding or limiting your exposure to those situations can help you control symptoms. For example, you may socialize mostly at home or in small groups, limit your time in crowded stores or go to restaurants at off-peak times. Also, many people with CFS and FM are selective about their exposure to television and movies, avoiding material that is emotionally arousing or has rapid scene changes. Some people have "media fasts," periods in which they watch no television, listen to no radio and ignore newspapers.

Some people with CFS and FM experience high levels of stress when they interact with people who are anxious, negative or demanding. Responses they have made include talking with the person, limiting contact, getting professional help, and ending the relationship. As one person wrote, "I have cut people out of my life that only irritate or don't support me. It was a hard thing to do but has made a big difference in how I feel."

Pacing, Order and Routine

Pacing strategies reduce stress. Reducing activity level, scheduling activity based on priorities, having short activity periods, scheduling important tasks for your best time of day, taking regular rests, and taking time for meditation or prayer all help control stress. As one person wrote, "I found that I could avoid much stress by knowing my limits. Planning too many activities in one day or scheduling them too close together are big stress triggers, so I try to prevent their activation by limiting the number of activities in a day and by giving myself plenty of time in between activities."

Another way to reduce stress is through routine: doing things in familiar ways and living your life according to a schedule reduces stress by reducing decision making and increasing predictability. It takes more energy to respond to a new situation than it does to something familiar, so by reducing the surprises and novelty in life, you reduce your stress.

Some people with CFS and FM create routine by living their lives according to a plan. By living their plan, they reduce the surprises and emotional shocks in their lives, and thereby reduce their stress. One wrote, "Up until two years ago my life had little routine in it and the result was frequent, lengthy crashes. My life was one big roller coaster. Now that I have a regular schedule, I can plan much better. Routine may sound boring, but it's a must for me." Another said, "Having a regular routine has been very useful, because having a predictable life has been the most effective way for me to reduce stress. A life with few surprises has reduced the pressure on me and given my body more time to heal."

References

Burns, David. *Feeling Good.* New York: Morrow, 1980.

Greenberger, Dennis and Christine Padesky. *Mind Over Mood: Change How You Feel by Changing the Way You Think.* New York: Guilford Press, 1995.

Hallowell, Edward. *Worry.* New York: Ballantine Books, 1997.

Seligman, Martin. *Learned Optimism.* New York: Knopf, 1991.

19. Addressing Feelings

Feelings such as sadness, worry, frustration and guilt are common and understandable responses to long-term illness. They are a reaction to the changes, limitations and uncertainty brought by illness. Because emotions are so common in long-term illness and so powerful, managing them deserves a place in your self-management plan.

There are two additional reasons to include managing emotions in your plan. First, CFS and fibromyalgia tend to make emotional reactions stronger than they were before and harder to control. The technical term is *labile*. People often say they cry more frequently, get upset more easily or have more angry outbursts than before they were ill. As one student in our program wrote, "Just recognizing that emotions are heightened as a result of CFS really helped me. Before learning that, I was quite puzzled by why I got upset about little things."

Second, feelings generated by being ill can create a vicious cycle. For example, being in constant pain can trigger worries about the future. Worry leads to muscle tension, which, in turn, increases pain. You can interrupt this cycle in several ways, such as by using relaxation to reduce muscle tension and by changing your "self-talk" to reduce worry.

The process by which feelings intensify symptoms occurs even with positive emotions, as suggested in a comment from another person in our program who said, "I cried at one of the classes because I was so happy to be around people who understood me. Almost immediately, I had an attack of brain fog." Any experience that triggers the production of adrenaline intensifies emotions and often makes symptoms worse as well.

Feelings, like other aspects of long-term illness, can be managed. Some strategies mentioned in earlier chapters may be useful for managing the emotions triggered by CFS and FM. For example, relaxation techniques can short-circuit the feedback effect in which symptoms and emotions reinforce one another. Also, changing your thinking using Cognitive Therapy may be help. This approach has been proven to be especially effective for treating anxiety and depression. Another general approach is to identify those situations (and sometimes people) that trigger strong emotions and plan a strategy of response ahead of time. Often, avoiding or minimizing stressful situations can reduce emotions.

In addition to self-help measures, the management of emotions can include professional help. Emotions such as depression and anxiety can be caused or intensified by changes in brain chemistry and may be treated using prescription anti-depressants or anti-anxiety medications. Also, counseling can be helpful. Talking with a therapist about the problems triggered by your illness does not imply that "it's all in your head." Rather, counseling offers help dealing with a difficult situation. The help may include support, suggestions of coping strategies and perspective on your situation. If you think talking with a counselor might be helpful, you might seek out one who specializes in treating people with long-term illness.

Depression

Depression is very common in people with CFS and fibromyalgia. This should not be surprising, given the effects of ongoing symptoms as well as the disruptions and uncertainty created by illness. Depression may be triggered by a sense of helplessness, by fear, frustration and anxiety, by loss, or by uncertainty about the future. Signs of depression include feelings of unhappiness or sadness, lack of interest in friends or activities, isolation, suicidal thoughts, and loss of self-esteem. Serious or long-term depression or thoughts of suicide call for immediate help from a doctor, therapist or suicide-prevention service.

There are two types of depression associated with CFS and fibromyalgia. One type is called situational depression, which means depression that occurs as a response to a particular set of circumstances, in this case having your life turned upside down by long-term illness. Self-management strategies such as those described below are usually helpful in response to this type of depression.

Depression may be biochemical as well, created by changes in the functioning of the brain. Prolonged stress may alter our biochemistry, causing depression. Self-management strategies may also be useful for this type of depression, but treatment normally includes medication as well.

Everyone has times when they feel unhappy or sad. We can recognize that these feelings are likely to occur from time to time and plan how to respond. (See box at end of this section for one person's planning strategies.) Here are a dozen strategies to consider for combating depression.

1. **Get Help.** If you are seriously depressed, suicidal or have been depressed for some time, get help now. Phone a suicide prevention center, talk to your doctor, see a psychologist or call a friend. If your situation is not urgent but depression reduces your ability to do your normal daily activities, you should consider professional help: counseling, medications or both. A therapist can provide an outside view of your situation, help you to accept your illness and support you

in your efforts to improve. If you have family tension because of illness, couples or family counseling can be helpful.

2. Get Active. Depression produces hopelessness, an attitude that becomes a self-fulfilling prophecy. Counteract those feelings by taking actions, such as those listed below, that have a good chance of helping. Being active changes mood; also, successes promote hope.

3. Establish Good Habits. Keeping to a daily routine regardless of how you feel can help counteract depression. Your daily round of activities will depend on the severity of your illness, and might include things like getting dressed, making the bed, cooking meals, taking a walk and watching a favorite TV program. Forcing yourself to do things, even if you don't want to, counteracts the inertia of depression.

4. Exercise. Exercise is a natural anti-depressant. It relieves tension, lessens stress and improves mood. Most exercise also involves being out of the house, thus bringing the added benefit of a change of scene. For ideas on how to exercise safely with CFS or FM, see Chapter 16.

5. Use Problem Solving. Taking action to solve a problem lifts the spirit as well as having practical benefits. Doing something counteracts the sense of helplessness, replacing it with a sense of control and accomplishment.

6. Rest. Some depression seems to be associated with physical symptoms, such as fatigue and pain. Resting to reduce these symptoms can also improve mood. One woman in our program described the connection by saying, "I can usually tell when I am doing more than my body can handle because I start to get depressed, not to mention short tempered and cranky. If I am well rested I am much happier."

7. Change Your Thinking. If you have a tendency to think of the worst that might happen, you can retrain yourself to speak soothingly and realistically when you're worried or depressed. For example, you can remind yourself that periods of bad feelings end. Change your mental climate by noticing what's going well and congratulating yourself on your accomplishments.

8. Do Something Pleasant. Pleasurable activities offer a distraction from symptoms and help create a good mood. The key is to find things that absorb your attention. Such activities might include reading, listening to music, sitting in the sun, taking a walk, doing crafts, solving puzzles, watching a movie and spending time with friends.

9. **Stay Connected.** Supportive human contact is very soothing. Calling a friend or getting together to talk, share a meal or see a movie counteracts isolation, preoccupation with problems and the low mood often associated with chronic illness. Just explaining yourself can give you perspective.

10. **Consider Medications.** If your depression is biochemical in origin, you may be helped by an anti-depressant medication. On the other hand, tranquilizers and narcotic painkillers intensify depression, so if you are depressed, it may be due partially to a medication side effect. If you suspect this, check with your doctor about a change of medication or a reduced dosage.

11. **Help Others.** Get involved with something larger than yourself to counteract isolation and preoccupation with self that often accompany illness and to rebuild self-esteem. Helping others might involve a regular commitment, like leading a support group, or something as simple as a phone call to an older relative, checking in with an old friend or trading favors.

12. **Manage Stress.** Controlling stress can help you manage your emotions, because stress tends to make emotions more intense. For ideas on managing stress, see Chapter 18 and the articles in the Stress Management archive of our website: *www.cfidsselfhelp.org*.

The Treasure Box and The 100 Hours Program: Two Anti-Depression Strategies

One person in our program has created two special anti-depression strategies. She calls one the Treasure Box of Pleasantries. It's a notebook containing compliments she has received, photos of places she has visited or would like to see, plus treasured notes, photos and cards. When her spirits are down, she picks them up by going through the box.

Her second strategy is the 100 Hours Program, a way to stay active and give herself a sense of purpose when her spirits are especially low. She scripts a period of up to 100 hours with "every special, pleasant and meaningful activity I can think of." Depending on her functional level, she might schedule hair and massage appointments or lunch with friends. In addition, she has a list of 50 activities she can do on her own. They include catching up on unread magazines, watching uplifting or interesting movies, perusing picture books and preparing easy-to-fix meals. Everything is worked into a schedule, which she keeps in a binder. She says that usually by the end of the time she is back to normal. The most important part is that "I don't have to think 'what do I do now'. I've planned it all out beforehand."

Anxiety and Worry

Anxiety and worry often accompany CFS and FM. The two conditions often create a loss of control over our bodies and over our ability to plan and predict. They also bring uncertainty about the future. We may be unclear about our prognosis and wonder whether we will improve and, if so, how much. We may worry about how far down we might slide and about becoming dependent or destitute.

Here are eight strategies that are often helpful in counteracting anxiety and worry. For more suggestions, see "Fifty Tips on the Management of Worry Without Using Medication" in the book *Worry* by Edward Hallowell.

1. **Practice Stress Reduction.** Learning relaxation and other stress reduction techniques can help reduce the intensity of your emotional reactions and, by doing so, reduce the echo effect in which emotions and symptoms amplify one another. A regular stress reduction practice can also lower "background worry," the ongoing anxiety that results from long-term stress. For instructions on several relaxation procedures, see the stress management section of our website: *www.cfidsselfhelp.org*.

2. **Use Problem Solving.** Taking action to solve a problem has a double payoff. You reduce or eliminate a practical concern that is bothering you and the process of taking action reduces anxiety.

3. **Change Your Thinking.** If you have a tendency to think of the worst that might happen, you can take steps to short-circuit the process in which your thoughts increase your anxiety. One antidote is to retrain yourself to speak soothingly when worried, saying things like "I've been here before and survived" or "this is probably not as bad as it seems." Also, you can do "reality checks" by testing your fears against facts and by asking for feedback from others. Learn to distinguish between toxic worry, which is unproductive and paralyzing, and good worry, which helps you plan. For more on changing thinking, see Chapter 31.

4. **Connect with Other People.** Feeling that you are part of something larger than yourself counteracts worry. Also, contact soothes worry, distracts you from preoccupation with problems, and provides reassurance.

5. **Exercise.** One of the best treatments for worry, exercise is both relaxing and distracting. For ideas about how to integrate exercise into your life when you have CFS or FM, see Chapter 16.

6. Pursue Pleasure. Reading, music, good conversation and other activities in which you can become immersed help change mood.

7. Don't Worry Alone. The act of sharing a worry almost always reduces its size and emotional weight. Discussion may help you find solutions and almost always makes the worry feel less threatening. Putting a worry into words translates it from the realm of imagination into something concrete and manageable. Seek out people who can offer support and reassurance.

8. Consider Counseling and Medications. Counseling and therapy can make worries more manageable. Also, just as drugs can help with depression, some people find that medications help them deal with anxiety. A drug will not be a complete solution to problems of anxiety, but it can be part of a comprehensive response.

A Note on Panic

About ten percent of people with CFS experience an especially severe and frightening form of fear called panic attacks. These are brief episodes of terror in which a person may feel he or she is about to die. Symptoms may include chest pain, heart palpitations and dizziness. In spite of overwhelming fear, people survive, but they may live a life of dread, apprehensive about when the next attack will occur. This kind of fear is treatable. For more, see the books by Edward Hallowell and Martin Seligman listed in the References at the end of the chapter.

Frustration and Anger

Frustration and anger are understandable reactions to chronic illness. Being sick is frustrating, since it brings uncertainty and loss of control. The frustrations of illness vary from not being able to plan daily activities to the loss of the future you had dreamed of. Further, irritability seems to be a symptom of CFS and fibromyalgia.

Self-management can make frustration manageable. The strategies described in earlier chapters, such as pacing and stress management, help reduce the sources of frustration. For example, by using pacing you can stabilize your life, reducing the swings between high symptoms and periods of remission, and reducing the occurrence of irritability. Stress reduction practices can help you relax, reducing your susceptibility to frustration. In both instances, techniques used for another purpose can reduce frustration as well.

Frustration can be destructive if it is expressed in a way that drives away people who want to help or those upon whom you depend. One way to respond positively is to create a situation focused on finding solutions to what is bothering you. If you are frustrated about a relationship, set up a conversation to discuss your problems. Pick a time to talk when you and the other person will be calm and not distracted.

Before the conversation, ask yourself what the other person could do to improve the situation. Then, when you meet, explain what is frustrating you. You may be able to defuse anger on the other side by stating that you realize that your illness is frustrating for everyone involved.

Here are six other strategies used by people in our program to deal with frustrations created by being ill. They focus on the goal of finding non-harmful ways to acknowledge and express anger.

1. **Get Support.** Expressing anger by talking it out with someone who is not the target of your frustration can release the feeling. As one student said, "The frustration and rage I felt about becoming ill has eased considerably since I joined a supportive group. I feel lucky to find a place to vent, be accepted and feel understood."

2. **Write.** Putting experience in words can be helpful. Psychologist James Pennebaker has found that people have fewer health problems if they write about traumatic events in a way that combines factual description and emotional reactions. (See his book *Opening Up* and also the article "Writing is Good Medicine" at *www.cfidsselfhelp.org.*) Verbalization of emotionally powerful experiences brings understanding. A related technique is to write a letter to the person you are mad at, and then tear it up instead of sending it.

3. **See Things from a Fresh Perspective.** The amount of anger you experience may be related to your thoughts, to how you see your situation. Imagine, for example, that you are waiting at a restaurant for a friend who is a half-hour late. You feel irritated. When the friend arrives, she reports that she was delayed because she was in an accident. Suddenly your emotion changes from anger to concern. Here's what one student said about the effects of seeing things in new ways: "I've learned to think about things in alternative ways. By taming my thoughts, I find that a lot of anger has disappeared and this is a most wonderful feeling. I have now reached the stage where most of this new thinking is automatic."

4. **Plan Your Response.** If you are irritated by comments like "I'm sure you would feel better if you would try this new remedy," you can prepare a response so that such comments don't bother you. In this case, you might say something like "Thanks for your suggestion, but I'm under my doctor's care and I'm following his treatment plan" or "I'll keep that in mind."

5. **Accept and Acknowledge the Feeling.** Some people report that they are able to dissipate the power of anger and other feelings by naming them. The exercise produces a detachment from the feeling. As one student said, "What seems to work for me is to think about the emotion I am having. If I am angry, I will say

'Ah, that is anger'. Then I say 'I accept this anger.' Then I describe the anger. Is it a huge anger or smoldering anger or little anger? Then I notice how it feels in my body."

6. **Get Professional Help.** Sometimes talking with a counselor can ease the pressures created by having a long-term illness. If frustration and anger are making your relationships more stressful, you might consider getting professional help. Look for a therapist who specializes in helping people with chronic illness.

Guilt

Guilt is another frequent companion of people with CFS and FM. Sometimes people blame themselves for becoming sick. At other times, guilt is triggered by the sense of not contributing to the family or to society. If you experience guilt, what can you do to ease the burden it imposes? Here are seven strategies to consider.

1. **Adjust Expectations.** Guilt is often triggered by a difference between a person's expectations and their capabilities. You can reduce guilt by adjusting your expectations downward to match your new level of functioning. As one person said, "I've lowered my standards for myself. This isn't easy, since I'm a recovering perfectionist." Another wrote that she tells herself, "If I were caring for an injured loved one, in distress, how would I take care of her? I should treat myself the same way."

2. **Reframe (Change Self-Talk).** Part of the process of adjustment is changing our internal dialogue or self-talk, so that it supports our efforts to live well with illness rather than generating guilt. One person says she has changed her self-talk about naps. In the past, when she took a nap, she told herself it was because she was lazy, but now she tells herself, "I am helping myself to be healthy. I am saving energy to spend time with my husband or to baby sit my grandchildren." Similarly, when feeling tired, you can say "This fatigue is not my fault; it came with CFS. So I don't need to feel guilty about not being able to do everything I used to." Or: "I didn't ask for FM, so why should I feel shame when it prevents me from doing things."

3. **Shift Attention.** Feeling guilty is inevitable, but we can control how we respond when feelings of guilt arise. One person said that she asks herself "Is this feeling productive?" In some cases, the answer will be "Yes." Guilt can draw our attention to ways in which we have failed to live up to our standards and can motivate us to act differently. (See next strategy.) If the feeling is not productive, however, it may be better to respond to guilt by turning our

attention elsewhere. As another person wrote, "It's better not to go some places in your head, so I've learned how to control my own thoughts."

4. **Apologize and Make Amends.** Guilt can be helpful if it motivates you to take better care of yourself in the future and to treat those around you with more consideration. One person said that if she does something to hurt her husband or her children, like lashing out at them verbally, she apologizes. Others say that they have used guilt over canceling out on commitments as an impetus to be more consistent in their pacing, making themselves more dependable.

5. **Educate Others.** Some guilt may be triggered by how others treat you. In addition to adjusting your expectations for yourself, you can work on changing the expectations others have of you as well. This involves educating the people in your life, emphasizing that CFS and FM are long-term conditions that impose significant limits and require adjustments of the person who is ill and those around her.

6. **Learn Assertiveness.** Another strategy for reducing guilt is to be assertive, standing up for yourself by stating what you will and won't do. One person in our program posts notes all over her house saying, "I'd love to but I just can't." The notes remind her what to say when people make requests. She says "seeing the notes so often ensures I remember to use this answer without feelings of guilt."

7. **Practice Relationship Triage.** A final strategy is to reevaluate your relationships, practicing what we call *relationship triage*: making explicit decisions about whom to include in your life, concentrating on the more valuable or necessary relationships and letting others go.

References

Hallowell, Edward. *Worry*. New York: Ballantine Books, 1997.

Pennebaker, James. *Opening Up: The Healing Power of Confiding in Others*. New York: Avon Books, 1990.

Seligman, Martin. *What You Can Change and What You Can't*. New York: Fawcett Columbine, 1993.

PART 5

Recast Relationships

20. Eight Ways to Improve Relationships

Serious illness creates stresses for most relationships. Relations with family, friends, coworkers and bosses, and even doctors are altered in ways that create new challenges for both people with CFS or FM and for those around them. People with CFS and FM experience many frustrations in their relationships.

- **Feeling Not Understood**: Other people may not believe you are ill or may not understand the seriousness of your condition.

- **Loss of Relationships**: Limitations and unpredictability of symptoms can make it difficult to maintain relationships. Some relationships may be lost, while others are redefined.

- **Guilt**: You may blame yourself for getting sick or for not contributing to family or society.

- **Feeling Undependable**: Unpredictability of symptoms often leads to cancelling out of commitments, creating misunderstanding and threatening some relationships.

- **Isolation**: You may feel a sense of isolation, either because of spending more time alone or because of feeling different from other people.

- **Fears of Dependency & Abandonment**: You may worry about losing your ability to care for yourself or fear that others upon whom you depend will leave you.

This chapter describes eight general strategies for improving relationships. Other chapters in this section focus on recasting family relationships, improving how couples work together, building a support network and working productively with doctors.

Assess & Triage

If you have CFS or FM, it is likely that many relationships will be redefined and some will end. You can make this transition a conscious and deliberate process by using *relationship triage*: making explicit decisions about whom to include in your support network.

One place to start your evaluation might be with the fact that CFS and fibromyalgia may make you feel more vulnerable to those who are negative or demanding. The cost of spending time with such people may be great enough to convince you that some relationships are not worth maintaining. You may decide to keep others and still others you may consider essential.

You might think of your relationships as a series of concentric rings. In this scheme, the inner ring contains the most important people in your life, typically family and closest friends. People on the outer ring are casual acquaintances. In between there may be one or two other rings of people with varying levels of importance. You may develop different approaches to people in various rings, concentrating on those in the inner ring.

The general idea is to concentrate on the more valuable or necessary relationships and letting others go. In the words of Dr. David Spiegel of Stanford: "Save your energy and use the illness as an excuse to disengage from unwanted social obligations. Simplify the relationships that are necessary but unrewarding, and eliminate the ones that are unnecessary *and* unrewarding."

Change How You Socialize

You may be able to preserve a good number of relationships by changing how you socialize. For example, if you have severe limits and cannot often get out of the house, you may be able to stay in touch with people using phone calls and emails, plus having people visit you.

Another adaptation is to limit the length of socializing, for example by limiting how long you talk on the phone or the amount of time you spend face-to-face with others. A third adaptation is to alter the settings in which you socialize. For example, you may be able to tolerate time in a restaurant if you go either before or after the busiest hours.

Other adjustments include limiting the number of people you socialize with and taking rest breaks. One woman with a large family told her adult children that she would not host more than one couple (and their children) at a time.

Do Your Part

CFS and FM alter the financial situations of many families, often force radical changes in how household tasks are divided up and reduce the number and scope of activities that families can do together. Just like you, your family members can feel isolated and helpless. They may experience loss because their dreams are put on hold. They may feel abandoned or frustrated by the restrictions on their lives. The unpredictability of symptoms can lead to others viewing you as undependable and mood swings can affect others as well.

One step toward easing strains in your relationships is to acknowledge that your illness creates problems for others. Your symptoms and moods, for example, may make you unpredictable, and your limits may force others to take on additional responsibilities. Express your appreciation for their efforts. Acknowledge that the illness can make you unreliable. Out of respect for other people, warn them that you might have to cancel on short notice. To help maintain the relationship, tell them that you value them and that canceling does not mean you don't like them.

Take responsibility for the problems your illness creates for others. For example, if your illness makes you moody, make a list of things you can do to help yourself feel better so that you avoid inflicting your moods on others. When you are feeling irritable, you might listen to music, take a walk or have a brief rest.

Change Expectations and Use Assertiveness

Because of guilt or pressure from others, you may do more than your body can tolerate. A solution is the combination of changing your expectations for yourself and being more assertive. Changing expectations is a gradual process by which you come to accept your limits and the need to adapt to a "new normal." For more, see Chapter 26.

Learning assertiveness can also be a gradual process, as you educate others about your limits. One part of assertiveness is to be very specific in the requests you make or limits you set. For example, say "Will you pick up bread and milk at the grocery store" or "I'd be glad to talk with you, but I'll only be good for 15 minutes." One person in our program communicates her envelope for the day to her family using a 1 to 10 scale. In her system, a 1 means "like I felt before I got sick" and 10 means "have to stay in bed all day." When asked to do something, she may respond by saying, "No, I can't do that; it's a 7 day."

Second, show that you understand the other person's situation. You might say something like, "I know my illness makes your life more difficult and that some things I say and do may be frustrating." Third, preface requests with a statement of appreciation, such as "I appreciate all you do for me." Fourth, if you find it difficult to be assertive, practice saying your request to yourself or someone you trust before making it to the person whose help you want.

Educate Others (Selectively)

Perhaps the most common relationship frustration among people with CFS and FM is not feeling understood and not being believed when we say we are ill. One response is to make efforts to educate others about CFS and FM. If you think educating others about your condition would make them more understanding or supportive, you might talk with them or give them something to read. The CFIDS Association of America has a pamphlet was "For Those Who Care" (*http://www.cfids.org/*) and we have similar materials in the Family and Friends section of our website: *http://www.cfidsselfhelp.org.*

A woman in our program was successful with a clever approach to sharing the CFIDS Association pamphlet. She gave copies to her husband and adult children, asking that they read it as their birthday present to her one year. Although the process took a full year, one by one her family members came to accept her CFS.

People report that educating others about CFS and FM often requires patience and is not always successful. Most who try eventually put limits on their efforts to educate others, focusing on the relationships that are most important and recognizing that some people may never understand or be sympathetic. One person reported that over time he has reduced his time talking to others about CFS, saying, "I still make efforts to educate, but I'm more selective about who I approach."

Your situation is different if you have school aged children. If they know you are sick, but don't understand your illness, they may fear that you will die or they may blame themselves for your suffering. By discussing your condition with them, they can replace fears with facts. Consider using the four guidelines offered by Dr. Julie Silver: 1) tell your children the name of your condition; 2) explain something about the illness (for example, that it is not thought to be contagious and is not anyone's fault); 3) describe the expected course of the illness (that it is likely to continue, but will be manageable); and 4) outline its effects and reassure them of your commitment to them (that you still love them despite being ill, and will do what you can, even though your activity level may be limited by the illness).

Build New Sources of Support

Creating new relationships can be a powerful antidote to frustration in relationships and can also counteract some of the losses and the isolation brought by illness. One good place to meet new friends is through support groups. (For ideas on locating a support group, see the chapter "Building a Support Network.") Similar experiences are available now on the Internet, at online chat rooms and message boards.

In thinking about how to meet your practical and emotional needs, consider putting together a group of people who can help. Some may offer practical help, such as grocery shopping, housecleaning or driving. Others may be companions for outings, such as a visit to a restaurant or a night at the movies. Still others may offer emotional support, by listening and offering reassurance. In any case, it's wise to have several people to fill these various needs, so that one or two people don't feel overburdened and burn out.

Professional support may be helpful as well. A sympathetic therapist can provide support and offer an outsider's view of your situation. If you're interested, you might look for one who specializes in working with people who have chronic illness. A local support group is often a good source of leads. Therapy can also be helpful for couples, offering a place in which the strains created by living with long-term illness can be addressed.

Accept Help and Help Others

Other people often feel helpless about our illness. By giving them something specific to do, you can do them a service while helping yourself. As one person in our program said, "People are often thrilled when I ask for help in clear, practical ways." A caution: asking too much of others in total or of one person in particular can risk caregiver burnout.

Helping others aids self-esteem. As one of our group leaders said, "Being a moderator helped me feel useful even when I was very ill and unable to accomplish much in the outside world." Doing things for others also gives others an incentive to stay in the relationship. As someone in our groups said, "I ask myself what I am doing to make a relationship valuable to the other person."

Embrace Solitude

Serious illness often forces people to spend much more time alone than before. A final strategy for responding to limits and the loss of relationships is to embrace solitude. Solitude can provide an opportunity to develop new solitary interests. Some patients, recognizing that they will be spending less time with people, have seen the situation as a chance to do things like reading and art work that they didn't have enough time for earlier in their lives. See, for example, JoWynn Johns' article "In Praise of Solitude," on our website.

References

Silver, Julie. "Chronic Pain in the Family," *Fibromyalgia Aware*: May 2005: 40-42.

Spiegel, David. *Living Beyond Limits*. New York: Times Books, 1993.

21. Family Issues

Chronic Fatigue Syndrome and fibromyalgia send shock waves through the family. Stress is increased, predictability is replaced with uncertainty, emotions are intensified and many practical aspects of life are altered. Issues that family members face include:

- Extra household tasks
- Extra childcare responsibilities
- Financial strains
- Caregiving responsibilities (for person with CFS or FM)
- Worry and uncertainty about the future
- Uncertainty about how to help the person who is ill
- Resentment and frustration
- Sadness and depression
- Increased stress
- Loss of companionship
- Sexual difficulties
- Strained communication
- Less socializing

Family adaptation focuses on the four issues described below. (Couples issues are explored in the next chapter.)

Redistributing Household Tasks

CFS and fibromyalgia usually lead to a redistribution of household tasks such as shopping, cooking, cleaning, laundry, bill paying and childcare. For those things the person with CFS or FM can't do or can't do in the same way as before, there are two main options: reassigning or simplifying.

Reassigning means finding someone else to do part or all of a task that the person who is ill used to do. Probably the most common solution is for the spouse to take over some or even many of the duties formerly done by the person who is ill. But there are other solutions as well. If there are children living at home, they may contribute in various ways, such as by keeping their rooms clean, helping with meal preparation and doing their own laundry. If adult children live nearby, they may offer practical help as well. Another solution is to pay for help, for example by hiring a cleaning service on an occasional or regular basis.

Simplifying means continuing to do something, but in a less elaborate or complete way. For example, people may clean house less often or cook less complicated meals. Some people simplify by downsizing their home, for example, by moving from a house to a condominium.

While accommodations to the CFS and FM are often required, the person who is ill may be able to increase the amount of work she does by using pacing. For example, several short periods of meal preparation with a break in between may allow someone with CFS/FM to make dinner without intensifying symptoms. The length of work periods may be increased by sitting rather than standing.

Also, by spreading housework over a week rather than doing it all at once, someone with CFS or FM can avoid the push and crash syndrome. Finally, most people with CFS or FM have good and bad times of day. It may be possible to get more done and avoid a flare up of symptoms by working during the good hours of the day.

Making Financial Adjustments

The financial effects of CFS and FM vary greatly. Some families make no changes to their finances or only minor adjustments. This may occur if the person who is ill was not employed when she or he became ill or was at or near retirement. Some people are able to arrange an early retirement with a reduced pension.

For other families, however, illness creates moderate to severe financial strain. If the person with CFS or FM is unable to work, family income may be reduced by half or more. A successful application for disability payments can reduce the deficit. (About one third of the people in our program report receiving disability benefits.)

In some cases, a healthy family member changes jobs to get work at higher pay or with better benefits. Some families establish financial discipline by using a budget and by reducing their spending. Others move to smaller, less costly homes, a strategy which can reduce both expenses and household tasks.

Social Adaptations

Because people with CFS and fibromyalgia have significantly less energy than before they were ill, they often reduce the time they spend with others, creating a loss of companionship both for themselves and for those around them. Factors such as energy limitations and sensitivity to sensory input (noise, light and movement) may force a reduction in the length, type or form of socializing. For example, a family may rent movies rather than going to a movie theater. In sum, CFS or FM may reduce the time a person can spend with family, lead to changes in setting, and force families to focus on less physically and mentally demanding activities.

Adjusting Expectations to a "New Normal"

Underlying the many practical adaptations described above is a psychological adjustment: acceptance that life has changed on a long-term basis. This is sometimes called finding a new normal and it involves coming to terms with loss. Family members lose some of the companionship they used to enjoy. They lose the future they envisioned for themselves and, like the person with CFS/FM, they are challenged to adjust to a different type of life than they had planned.

Coming to terms with loss and adapting to a new life usually takes several years to a decade. The end point of this process is acceptance, a complex attitude that includes recognizing that life has changed, accepting the limitations imposed by illness and adjusting expectations to match new capabilities. Acceptance does not mean resignation, but rather a commitment to live the best life possible under the circumstances, recognizing that it will be a different kind of life than before. People in our program and their families report using three strategies to build a new life:

1. **Adjust Goals to Fit Abilities.** Focus on those things that are still possible, rather than on those that are no longer possible. This is sometimes called adjusting expectations or reframing your experience.

2. **Develop New Interests.** A powerful antidote to loss is to develop new interests and, from that, a new sense of purpose and meaning. A couple, in which the wife is housebound, have taken up the study of music using a course on DVD. The project is a shared activity that replaces those lost to illness.

3. **Finding Positive Models.** People often report that their adjustment to CFS/FM was accelerated once they found other patients who had adapted successfully. Families can follow the same approach, seeking out other families who can provide both practical ideas and models of successful adaptation.

22. Couples Issues

CFS and fibromyalgia put couples under stress. This chapter offers strategies for addressing three problems faced by couples: sexual difficulties, strained communication and caregiver burnout.

Improving Intimacy

When CFS or fibromyalgia enters a marriage, one casualty can be intimacy between the partners. Pain, reduced energy, reduced interest, health problems of the partner, and increased responsibilities for the healthy spouse can all affect a couple's sex life, but, like other aspects of long-term illness, intimacy problems can be addressed as well.

When we asked people in our program to describe the effects of their illness on their sexuality, all those who responded said that illness had reduced their sexual activity. Many people mentioned having a much lower level of sexual desire than before, due to factors like ongoing fatigue and pain, and the side effects of medications. Other causes of sexual problems included the effects of menopause, relationship strains, and the medical problems and/or impotence of their partner.

Even though people said that they had either reduced their sexual expression or given up sex, most also reported using a variety of strategies that have either enabled them to adapt their sexual life to their illness or to connect with their partner in other ways. Here are six of the most common adaptations.

1. **Talking.** Several people reported that their relationship with their partner improved after they talked openly about their reduced interest in sex. As one said, "I explained that I still loved him and felt the same (or more strongly) about him, but I just couldn't show that through initiating sex...I have no desire for self-pleasure either. Explaining that sure made a difference to his acceptance of my state!" Others reported that they benefited from open communication in bed. One said, "I let him know if a certain position hurts and we change positions."

2. Alternative Activities. Another very common theme was adapting to illness by focusing on alternatives to conventional sex. One person wrote, "The times I am not up to having intercourse, he knows I am usually up for some cuddling and happy to satisfy him another way." Others wrote of alternatives to intercourse, for those who think that appropriate. "You don't have to have intercourse to be sexually connected...You can be satisfied by manual stimulation and also oral sex."

Others have found other ways to express their affection: through hugging, kissing, and holding hands, through words of appreciation and thoughtful acts, and through shared activities like going out for dinner together, watching a favorite TV program or giving one another a massage. One said, "We still hug, kiss and say 'I love you' lots. I feel we have a very strong and healthy relationship."

3. Planning. A third common adaptation is planning for sex. Several people mentioned taking extra rest or reducing their activity level on days they anticipated having sex. Also, a number said they and their partners plan "dates." One said, "What my husband and I have learned is that we need to schedule a 'date'. I actually put it on my calendar." Another said, "The 'date' planning has worked for me because I tend to do less of the things that I know will cause me residual pain."

Others mentioned being mindful of time of day. Pain and other symptoms may be lower during certain hours of the day. By timing intimacy for those times, couples minimize discomfort and increase enjoyment.

Another couple reported increasing the frequency of sex through making a commitment to having sex once a week. The wife reported that more frequent encounters made sex less painful and her husband "is much more cheerful and doing more around the house."

4. Flexibility and Experimentation. Given the often unpredictable course of CFS and FM, it can help to be flexible about when sex occurs and what positions and activities are involved. One person said, "We've experimented with timing (morning is best), position (I seem to do best on my side) and lubricants." Others use observation as a basis for experimentation. One person wrote, "I noticed that in the summer I had more desire and realized it had to do with the heat, so we started to shower together."

5. Addressing Pain and Hormone Problems. Some people said that their sex lives improved after treatment of pain and hormone problems. They reported treating pain by the use of pain pills, topical ointments, massage and heat, and by adapting how intimacy occurs.

There are several factors involved in the use of medication. One solution is for the person who is ill to time the taking of pain medication so that it will be at peak effectiveness when sex is planned to occur. The type of pain medication is also important. The person with pain may want to avoid narcotic pain medications and tranquilizers, which dull the senses as well as reducing pain. Other means of pain reduction include taking a bath before sex, stretching and massage.

Pain can be reduced by using positions that are comfortable, by changing positions periodically during intimacy and by alternating activity and rest. Another pain control approach is the combination of distraction and meditation. Distraction means reducing pain by placing attention elsewhere, focusing on sensations, both those given and those received. Also, concentrating on mental images of making love keeps the mind focused on pleasure, distracting attention from pain.

Several people in our groups also commented on how their interest in sex had improved with hormone treatment, either estrogen, testosterone or both. One said that testing showed that both her estrogen and testosterone levels were low. Treatment of the latter "not only helped libido, but my energy level as well." Hormone problems can also affect men.

6. **Emphasis on Caring.** A number of people distinguished between intimacy and sex, and said they and their partners focused on closeness and mutual caring. One wrote, "Sex is important in a relationship, but I don't feel that it is the most important. I think all of the little everyday things that we do for each other and being supportive of each other is what really makes a marriage."

Another said, "My husband and I have found we don't NEED to express our affection sexually...For us, sex does not compare to the kind of fulfillment which is a beautiful thing when shared between two people who are filled with warm, tender, loving feelings toward each other." She wrote of expressing affection through sharing time together, touching, caressing, and cuddling.

CFS or fibromyalgia do not have to mean the end of sex. Using flexibility, experimentation and good communication, couples can continue to enjoy sex and may be able to strengthen their relationship. For those who decide that sex will no longer be a part of their relationship, a focus on other aspects of the relationship can foster closeness.

Improving Communication

The stresses brought by serious illness can make good communication difficult. To complicate matters, some may experience cognitive problems. Here are seven ideas for how to improve communication if you or your partner have CFS or FM.

1. **Pick a Good Time and Setting.** If you have something important to discuss with a significant person in your life, select a time when both of you will be at your best. It should be a time when both of you can give good attention and you will not be distracted by pain or brain fog, preferably during your best hours of the day. Choose a place that minimizes distractions and interruptions.

2. **Practice Good Listening Skills.** Good communication is based on each person understanding the other person's views. Understanding begins with listening, which means focusing your attention on what is being said, with the goal of understanding the speaker's point of view.

   Listening works best if it occurs without interruption. After the person is finished speaking, respond by acknowledging having heard them. You might say something as simple as, "I understand." If you are not clear, you can respond by asking for clarification or more information. You might say something like, "I'm not sure I understand. Can you say something more?"

   From time to time, check whether you have understood the other person's position by restating it in your own words. You could say, "Let me try to summarize what I've heard and you can tell me if I'm understanding you."

3. **Focus on One Thing at a Time and Be Specific.** Focus on one issue at a time. If you are requesting that the other person change, be specific in your request. Avoid making general requests such as, "I need help with the housework." The person being asked may wonder what would be involved in responding to the request. Instead, say something like, "Can you do a load of laundry today?" or "Can you do the grocery shopping?"

   If you are the one being asked to do something, it's reasonable to defer giving a yes or no answer until you are confident you understand what is expected of you. You can ask, "What specifically would you like me to do?" Even if you decide to decline, you can still acknowledge the importance of the request to the person asking for help.

4. **Aim for Solutions.** Have as your goal finding solutions, not blaming one another or finding fault. The idea is to be able to discuss problems in a constructive rather than a confrontational way. Treat each other with respect, acknowledging his or her support and effort. Avoid demeaning comments, sarcasm and blaming. Acknowledge your part in shared problems and express appreciation for the other's efforts.

5. **Use Problem Solving.** Use problem solving to find solutions. Begin by brainstorming, which means thinking of a variety of possible ways to solve a problem. In brainstorming, the goal is to generate as many ideas as possible, without evaluating them. For example, if your problem is how to do household

chores when one member of the family is ill, alternatives might include dividing up the chores differently among members of the family, hiring occasional or regular assistance, simplifying tasks (for example, having simpler meals or cleaning less frequently), and moving to a smaller home that is easier to maintain.

Second, you evaluate each proposed solution, decide which ones are most promising and try one or two of them. Third, after giving each solution a fair try, evaluate the results. Some potential remedies may not work, so you may need to have further discussions and try other solutions. The final solution may be a combination of several approaches. If several strategies are unsuccessful, you may decide that a problem may not be solvable or not solvable at the present time.

6. Consider Getting Help. In many cases, you will be able to solve your problems yourself, but at times you may want to get help, either in understanding the causes of your problem or in finding solutions. So it may help to ask what resources are available to you. For example, to get a fresh perspective on your situation, you might ask other families how they have solved a similar problem or you might ask what community resources (church and public groups) are available.

Also, if conversations about your problems are not productive, you can consider getting professional help. A counselor can facilitate a solution to particular problems and also help you practice good problem solving skills.

7. Have Regular Relationship Discussions. Finally, here's a technique that one couple in our program uses to nurture their relationship and to solve problems in their lives: having regular discussions of their relationship. They set aside Sunday evenings as a time to discuss any issue that is on their minds, calling it their "talk night."

Having regular discussions means that both husband and wife know that they have a forum in which to state problems and frustrations, and a means for finding solutions. Also, because the talks are frequent, they can refine their communication skills through regular practice.

The husband explains that "Anything either of us sees as a problem or causing stress is a likely topic. Even very minor things are OK." Topics include an issue one has with the other, problems with friends or children or problems around the house. "A rule is that we each openly listen to the other without being defensive. We problem-solve together to come up with a resolution for each issue. After doing talk night we start each week refreshed and with the feeling that comes from having dealt with whatever problems were there."

Tips for the Caregiver

Caring for someone with CFS or FM can be a stressful experience. You may take on extra responsibilities, experience financial strain, feel frustrated and resentful at times, lose companionship, face uncertainty about the future, and experience both reduced socializing and sexual difficulties. Even with all the challenges brought by serious illness, there are many ways to take care of yourself. Here are nine to consider.

1. **Maintain Your Health.** This is the number 1 recommendation of experts on caregiving. To serve your loved one well and to avoid resentment and burnout, take time to get adequate rest, to eat well and to exercise.

2. **Accept Help.** When people offer to help, accept the offer and suggest specific things that they can do. If your finances allow, consider paying for help in such areas as meals, housecleaning and transportation.

3. **Take Time for Yourself.** Get a respite from caregiving by spending time away from the person who is ill, for example by pursuing a hobby. Give yourself an opportunity for leisure and enjoyment, a way to recharge your batteries.

4. **Educate Yourself.** Seek information about CFS or FM, especially strategies for reducing symptoms and improving quality of life. One source is the articles on our website: *www.cfidsselfhelp.org*. See the article "Educate Yourself" for a list of patient organizations, other websites and books about the two conditions.

5. **Stay Connected.** Avoid isolation and reduce stress by maintaining relationships with extended family and friends. This may mean getting together regularly for exercise or outings with friends, spending time with children or any other kind of socializing that keeps you connected with others.

6. **Consider Counseling.** Be sensitive to signs of stress and consider seeing a counselor if you detect them. Signs that counseling might be appropriate include feeling exhausted, depressed or burned out, or over-reacting, such as by angry outbursts. Counseling can be helpful for gaining perspective on your situation or to explore communication problems. You might get help in individual sessions or in joint sessions with the person who is ill.

7. **Grieve Your Losses.** Just as people with CFS and FM experience many losses, so do those around them. They are deprived of part of the companionship the patient used to provide, as well as her work around the house and, in many cases, financial contribution. And, just as the person who is ill has lost the

future she hoped for, so do you have to adjust your dreams for the future. Like the person in your life with CFS and FM, you, too, need to grieve your losses. For ideas on how to work through loss, see the discussion of finding a "new normal" in the previous chapter and also Chapter 26.

8. Create New Shared Activities. Serious illness may make it impossible for you to spend time with the person who is ill in the same way as before, but you can develop new shared activities to do together. One couple told us they took up the study of music using courses on DVD. The husband in another couple said that once he realized his wife's new limits, they shifted from camping and hiking to dinner and a movie.

The point is to create occasions for shared pleasure, so that the relationship is strengthened and both ill and healthy members of the family don't come to see their relationships as just about illness and deprivation.

9. Seek Support from Other Caregivers. Fellow caregivers can offer strength, support, inspiration and models of successful adaptation. You might meet such people through patient support groups.

23. How Family and Friends Can Help

Family members and friends can help people with CFS or FM in many ways. Some help is practical, such as taking on tasks the person with CFS or FM is no longer able to do or providing transportation to medical visits. Some help is emotional, offering a listening ear or some reassurance.

But perhaps the biggest aid is supporting the person with CFS or FM in her efforts to adjust her life to the limits imposed by long-term illness. The severity of symptoms and sometimes even the course of a person's illness are affected by how she lives her day to day life. If you are a family member or friend of someone with CFS or FM, the way you interact with that person will have a significant effect on her, helping her gain control over her condition or making that goal more difficult. Here's how you can help in five important areas.

Activity Limits and Pacing

Probably the single most important lifestyle change for controlling symptoms is to adjust activity level to fit the limits imposed by illness. This approach is often called pacing. In contrast to fighting the body with repeated cycles of push and crash, the person who adapts to limits seeks to understand the body's new requirements and to live within them. Pacing, above all, means reducing one's overall activity level. The reduction varies depending on the severity of symptoms, but is usually between 50% and 80%. The average person in our program rates herself at 30 or 35 on the CFS/FM Rating Scale found in Chapter 2, which allows for about three hours of activity a day.

Family and friends can help the person with CFS or FM to adapt by accepting that she can do less than before and by acknowledging that she will need to spend more time in rest and do things in new ways (such as alternating activity and rest).

Improving Sleep

Poor sleep is one of the most common and troublesome issues in both CFS and fibromyalgia. Treatment of sleep problems often includes prescription medications, but lifestyle changes can also be useful. Sleep can be improved by having an environment conducive to sleep and by having good sleep habits, such as a regular time to go to bed each night.

A comfortable sleep environment includes a good mattress and control of light, noise and temperature. (Noise includes snoring.) Some couples solve noise problems by sleeping in separate rooms. This strategy also allows the person who is ill to have greater control over other elements in the sleep environment.

Fighting the Fog

Most people with CFS and fibromyalgia experience cognitive difficulties, often called "brain fog" or "fibro fog." These problems include confusion, difficulty concentrating, fumbling for words and lapses in short-term memory. Family members can help the person with CFS/FM reduce the amount and the effects of cognitive problems by supporting their loved one in her efforts to control fog.

One common technique for combatting fog is the use of lists and other reminders. People with CFS and FM often post notes to themselves in places like the refrigerator, bathroom mirror or the inside of the front door.

Most people with CFS and fibromyalgia feel confused by sensory input coming from several sources at one time. They are likely to think more clearly if noise and light are at levels they can tolerate, and if sensory data is limited to one source at a time. Another way to limit sensory overload is to have an orderly physical environment, so reducing clutter is helpful. A related strategy is to live a predictable life using routines. For example, always putting keys in the same place and having meals at the same time every day.

A final strategy for reducing the effects of brain fog is to be sensitive to time of day. Most people with CFS and FM have better and worse periods during the day and may be able to get much more done if they schedule activity for good hours of the day.

Sensitivity to Stress

Stress is a challenge for everyone, but it is especially difficult for people with CFS and FM. The two conditions add new stressors and also make people more vulnerable to stress. CFS and FM reset people's "stress thermostat," so that the effects of a given level of stress are greater than they would be for a healthy person. The combination of additional stressors and increased vulnerability creates a double challenge. Stress is multiplied at the same time that stress takes a greater toll.

One of the best stress management strategies is preventive: minimizing the body's stress response by avoiding stressful situations. This can include a person's avoiding foods and other substances to which they are allergic, minimizing situations that create sensory overload (for example, crowds and noisy places) and limiting contact with anxious or negative people. Another stress avoidance technique is routine: doing things in familiar ways and living life according to a schedule.

Special Events

Special events, such as vacations, holiday celebrations or (for some people) having people over for dinner, require special measures. As non-routine events, they require more energy than everyday life and can easily lead to a relapse. Family members and friends can help by supporting the person with CFS or FM in her use of strategies that reduce the cost of a special event.

The most effective strategy is to take more rest than usual, before, during and after a special event, storing up energy by taking extra rest before the event, limiting symptoms by taking extra rest during and taking whatever extra rest is needed afterwards.

Patients often minimize the cost of a special event by changing their role or level of involvement. They might stop cooking the meal for a holiday celebration and instead ask family members to bring one dish each. Or they might go to event, but stay for less time than when they were healthy or change their level of involvement based on symptoms. On a trip, for example, they might opt out of some activities in order to take additional rest.

24. Building a Support Network

Whether you live with family or alone, having a support network is one of the key ingredients to living well with a long-term illness.

Support can take many forms. One type is practical help, such as grocery shopping, housecleaning or driving. A second type is companionship for activities, such as someone to go to a movie with. A third type is acceptance, feeling believed when you say you are ill. And a final type is understanding, the sense that others know what you are going through.

Family relations can meet support needs in varying degrees, but usually do not provide people with all the support they would like. Connecting with people beyond the family opens up new opportunities while reducing the burden on those closest at hand. If you live on your own, building a support network is all the more crucial.

Your Support Network

In thinking about how to meet your practical and emotional needs, consider putting together a network of people who can help. In *Fibromyalgia & Chronic Myofascial Pain: A Survival Manual,* Devin Starlanyl and Mary Ellen Copeland suggest that such a network contain at least five people. Some may offer practical help. Others may help you meet your needs for socializing. Still others may offer emotional support by listening and offering reassurance or insight. Avoid over-burdening and burn-out by having a pool of several people to fill these needs.

A Coach

It can be especially helpful to have one person to whom you can turn for emotional support and an objective view of your life. That person could be your spouse, a good friend, someone else with CFS/FM or a counselor. People in our program have said that their spouse often functions in this way: reminding them of their limits, encouraging them when they are feeling down and suggesting new strategies they can try.

Support Groups & Classes

Contact with other people who have CFS or FM can counteract isolation and provide an experience of being acknowledged and supported. Such contact can be a way to feel understood, comforted and inspired.

Support groups and classes such as ours are one way to meet fellow patients. In addition to connecting with others who have CFS/FM, support groups can provide information, such as names of local doctors who treat CFS and fibromyalgia. Also, groups offer a way to be helpful, thus counteracting the loss of self-esteem that often results from serious illness. And, finally, they can offer models of successful coping, thus dispelling fear. Similar experiences are available now on the Internet, at online chat rooms and message boards.

While support groups can be helpful, not all provide a positive experience. Some groups are negative in tone, reinforcing a sense of victimhood. Some groups are dominated by one or a few people. Others focus on responding positively to illness and insure participation from all members who wish to speak.

Contact with fellow patients in a group setting can be very powerful and may leave you feeling upset at times. When such contact is negative, it can reinforce isolation and powerlessness. In a supportive group, however, the discomfort should be followed by a new perspective on your situation and increased confidence about your ability to manage the illness.

I suggest you evaluate support groups based on the effects they have on you. A helpful group is one in which you feel a sense of belonging, which gives you something positive to take home, either inspiration or practical tips, and which offers models of living successfully with illness.

Finding Support Groups

The CFIDS Association of America maintains a state-by-state list of CFS support groups in the United States. They will mail a list of groups in your state at no cost. (You can contact them at 704/365-2343 or via their website: *http://www.cfids.org/*.)

For lists of FM support groups, see the website of the National Fibromyalgia Association (*http://www.fmaware.org/*) and also the ProHealth website (*http://www. prohealth.com/supportgroups/*), which also has listings for CFS groups. If you are looking for ideas on how to manage your illness more effectively, you might consider self-help classes for people with CFS and fibromyalgia, which include our online courses. (See our website: *www.cfidsselfhelp.org*.)

Professional Support

Another kind of support is the professional help offered by counselors and psychotherapists. A sympathetic therapist can offer encouragement, provide an outsider's view of your situation and give you continuity. If you're interested, you might look for one who specializes in working with people who have chronic illness. A support group can be a good source of leads. Therapy can also be helpful for couples, offering a place in which the strains created by living with long-term illness can be explored and solutions worked out.

25. Finding and Working with Doctors

With a long-term illness, you have a different role with health care providers than is typical for acute illnesses. Because your condition is an ongoing one, and you are the day-to-day manager, the patient/provider relationship is more appropriately a partnership in which you play an active role, selecting the members of your health care team and working with them to improve your quality of life.

It is reasonable for you to expect some things of the people helping you. They should know about your illness or be willing to learn about it. They should believe your illness is real, treat you with respect and be willing to experiment to find treatments that work in your individual circumstances. Looking at the relationship from the other side, you should have realistic expectations of your providers. Since there is so far no cure for either CFS or FM, it is appropriate to focus on treating symptoms to improve your quality of life. Since there are no medical treatments that are consistently helpful for people with CFS and FM, you will probably have to try several to many to find what works for you.

For Dr. Lapp's thoughts on this topic, see his article "How Your Doctor Can Help If You Have CFS/ME" at *www.cfidsselfhelp.org*. Dr. Lapp is director of the Hunter-Hopkins Center in Charlotte, North Carolina, a clinic that specializes in treating CFS and FM.

Sources of Help

Given the complexity of chronic illness and the likelihood of having several medical problems, you may well want to assemble a group of providers to help you live better. You will need to explain your situation and special needs to all of them.

1. **Physicians.** Medical doctors often seen by CFS and fibromyalgia patients include both primary care physicians and specialists. Among the latter are rheumatologists (doctors who specialize in arthritis and related illnesses, including fibromyalgia), psychiatrists (doctors who specialize in mental and emotional problems and who prescribe medications for problems like anxiety and depression), doctors who specialize in pain management and doctors who treat sleep disorders.

2. **Other Medical Providers.** Doctors may refer you to physical or occupational therapists, who can help you address problems through physical manipulation, exercise training and adjustments to daily activities. You can get spinal adjustments from chiropractors.

3. **Other Sources of Help.** You can receive help with emotional problems triggered by long-term illness from psychologists and therapists. They work both with individual patients and with families. Massage therapists provide relief with hands-on treatment. Nutritionists address problems with nutrition and food allergies. You may also get help from teachers and group leaders if you join exercise programs or take classes in subjects like yoga or Tai Chi. Lastly, fellow patients can provide support, understanding and inspiration.

Finding a Doctor

You can be forgiven if you are frustrated about finding sensitive and appropriate medical care. Studies suggest that it typically takes several years to receive a diagnosis of CFS or fibromyalgia, a period in which people are often dismissed and their complaints ignored. I would encourage you to persevere in your search for doctors who believe you when you say you are sick and who treat you with respect. In our experience, people with CFS and fibromyalgia who have sought sympathetic and knowledgeable physicians have usually found them.

How do you find a doctor who is knowledgeable and whom you trust? One good starting point is referrals from fellow patients. Support groups are often a good way to meet other patients. The CFIDS Association of America maintains a state-by-state list of CFS support groups in the United States. They will mail a list of groups in your state at no cost. (You can contact them at 704/365-2343 or through their website: *www.cfids.org* .) Some local chapters of the Arthritis Foundation (*www.arthritis.org*) provide physician referrals for FM. For lists of FM support groups, see the ProHealth and National Fibromyalgia Association websites (*http://www.prohealth.com/supportgroups/* and *www.fmaware.org*).

Other resources for finding doctors include:

- Fibromyalgia Network (*www.fmnetnews.com*)
- Good Doctor list at Co-Cure (*www.co-cure.org/Good-Doc.htm*)
- FMS Community website (*www.fmscommunity.org/findingadoctor.htm*)
- Devin Starlanyl's site (*www.sover.net/~devstar/provider.htm*).

Visits

Your doctor and other health care providers are important allies in your effort to live well with your illness. This section contains some suggestions for making these relationships productive. I'll focus on the doctor/patient relationship, but the principles apply to most of the other providers as well.

Because you have a long-term condition, you have the opportunity to establish long-term relationships with your physicians. As with other significant relationships, you should feel comfortable expressing your ideas and discussing alternatives. You should also be able to negotiate a treatment plan acceptable to both of you. Because there are no standard treatments for either CFS or fibromyalgia, and because treatments may be effective for only a period of time, you and your physicians should agree that treatment will consist of experiments. Some of the experiments may work; some probably won't; and others will work, but only for a while.

If you have found physicians who are supportive, who want to help you feel better and who are willing to experiment to find which treatments help you, the biggest obstacle to a good relationship is time. Particularly today, doctors work on a tight schedule that often leaves them as frustrated as patients. By viewing your visits with them as professional meetings, you can structure your time productively. One way to make your visits productive is by "taking P.A.R.T." The letters mean Prepare, be Active, Repeat, and Take action. (This acronym is adapted from advice about doctor/patient relationships in *The Arthritis Helpbook.*)

Prepare

Prepare for the visit by asking yourself why you are going and what you expect from the doctor. Make a list of your questions or concerns. Are you worried about a new symptom? Would you like a new medication? Do you want the doctor to submit a document supporting a disability claim? Write down your concerns, recognizing that probably no more than two or three issues will be addressed in one visit.

As part of your preparation, consider rehearsing a concise description of your symptoms and situation. Studies suggest that doctors allow around 20 seconds for a patient to describe her concerns before interrupting, so be prepared to state succinctly your concerns and what you want from the doctor. Describe your problems and goals concretely, so the doctor knows they are manageable within the constraints of the appointment.

Your opening statement might include when your symptoms started, where they are located and what changes in your life might account for them. Also, consider reporting on previous treatments, such as the effectiveness and side effects of a medication. If you are uncertain about whether you can explain yourself adequately or remember the doctor's response, you might ask a family member or friend to accompany you.

Be Active

Take an active role in your appointment. Begin the visit by describing briefly your main concerns, as described above. You might say something like, "I came in to talk about improving my sleep. I've been having trouble falling asleep; I wake up several times during the night, and the drug I've been taking doesn't seem to be effective any more." You may want to include a reference to your thoughts and feelings about the problem. For example, if sleep is your problem, you might say, "I'm concerned because I've been doing better overall and I'm afraid that poor sleep may make all my other symptoms worse and I'll be back where I was two years ago." If you have a written list of concerns, give it to the doctor.

In addition to making a clear and concise statement of your concerns, take an active role in the meeting by interacting with the doctor. If you don't understand something, ask her to explain it again. If you think a proposed treatment won't work or you are unwilling to try it, tell the doctor. If your insurance doesn't cover all the proposed treatments, make your financial constraints known. If the doctor suggests a medication, ask:

- How and when should I take it, and for how long?
- How soon will the effects appear?
- What are the most common side effects and what should I do about them?
- What are my other options?
- How and when should I report to you about my experience with the drug?

Repeat

To check your understanding, repeat back to the doctor the key points she has made. For example, you might state that you understand the doctor is recommending you treat your sleep problem by taking two medications, one to help you fall asleep and the other to help you stay asleep.

If you don't understand or are not clear, ask the doctor to repeat. The purpose of repeating is to make sure that you and the doctor have a common understanding of the discussion and to clear up misunderstandings of the diagnosis and of the steps you will take after the visit.

Take Action

As the visit is ending, make sure you are clear about what you are expected to do as a result of the appointment. Imagine that you are back home and want to follow-up on the visit: do you have all the information you need and do you understand what the doctor has asked you to do?

If you discussed a medication, did you receive a prescription? If so, do you understand how long you will take the drug, how many times a day and at what hours to take it, and what kind of side effects to expect? What about follow-up? Does the doctor want you to return? If so, how soon? Is it OK to check in by phone or to contact her only if you have a problem? If you are not clear about what you should do as a result of the visit, or you are not certain you can remember, write down the doctor's instructions or ask the doctor to do so.

PART 6

Move From Loss to Hope

26. Grieving Your Losses

Coming to terms with loss is one of the biggest challenges of CFS and fibromyalgia. Both conditions create many serious losses, including loss of control over one's body, loss of friends and loss of valued activities. People are often forced to give up their job and so lose income, companionship and challenge. And often people have to abandon dreams, thus losing the future they had envisioned for themselves. In sum, we experience the loss of the person we used to be and the person we hoped to become.

The pervasiveness of loss presents us with some of our most daunting tasks: keeping hope alive and bringing new meaning to life when much has been taken away. This chapter discusses how to work through loss. The next chapter describes how to move beyond loss to build a new life.

Responses to Loss

Loss triggers the emotional reaction known as grief. While grief is usually associated with the death of a loved one, it can occur after any loss. Responses to loss are sometimes discussed in terms of the well-known stages of death described by Elizabeth Kubler-Ross in her book *On Death and Dying*: denial, anger, bargaining, depression and acceptance. For most people, however, there is not a neat, orderly progression implied by the term stages. Rather, grief is a more individual process in which a person may experience some, but not necessarily all, of the emotions described by Kubler-Ross. Also, a person may experience some emotions more than once or may feel two or more at the same time.

Working through grief can produce a double benefit. Not only will you resolve a key psychological issue, you may also help yourself physically as well. Grieving is associated with the flare-up of symptoms, so resolving feelings of loss can help control symptoms. The health effects of working through grief were shown in a study of HIV-positive men who had lost a close friend to AIDS. The research found that those men who were able to find meaning in the loss had a significantly lower risk of dying of AIDS themselves in the following several years.

Denial and Disbelief

A diagnosis of CFS or fibromyalgia often produces relief by giving a name to suffering, but this initial reaction may be accompanied by shock and disbelief. A diagnosis of either CFS or FM means being told you have a condition for which there is no cure and which has no consistently effective medical treatments. Common reactions include ignoring the diagnosis by continuing to lead a busy life or seeking a cure by going from doctor to doctor or by trying special treatments or diets.

Denial can be an adaptive response, allowing you to adjust gradually to all that is different and to the uncertainty brought by the illness. Denial is a way to keep hope alive after being told that your life has changed and may never be the same. But, if you get stuck in this reaction, you won't be able to face your situation realistically. The repeated unsuccessful attempts at a miracle cure may reinforce a sense of helplessness and despair. Gaining some control over symptoms and using self-management strategies, such as pacing and stress reduction, can replace the sense of helplessness with experiences of control.

Fear and Worry

Fear and worry are common reactions to the unpredictability and uncertainty brought by illness. Not knowing what the future holds and the sense that your life is out of control can both produce tremendous anxiety.

Developing and implementing a self-management plan can address worry in several ways. First, the use of pacing, often in combination with medications, can bring stability, thereby replacing uncertainty with predictability. Second, because fear is usually accompanied by muscle tension, you can break the connection between emotion and physical reaction by including relaxation procedures in your plan. Third, because anxiety usually produces negative thoughts, being attentive to self-talk and changing it to be less fearful and more realistic reduces anxiety. (For more on self-talk, see Chapter 31.) Fourth, educating yourself about your illness can help by replacing worries with facts. For example, some fears about the future may be alleviated by knowing that neither CFS nor fibromyalgia is usually progressive and that many people with CFS and FM improve. (For more strategies, see the discussion of anxiety and worry in Chapter 19.)

Frustration and Anger

Frustration and anger are common reactions to loss and the experience of having your life changed by something over which you had no control. They are honest emotions that honor the recognition that life changed for no apparent reason, becoming much more difficult. Frustration can also be triggered by the experience of uncertainty.

Feeling angry is normal and can have positive effects if it motivates you to work to regain control of your life or if it moves you to channel your energy to help others. But anger can be destructive if it is expressed in a way that drives away people who want to help or on whom you depend. Expressing anger by blowing up, shouting or by being cruel is hurtful. Resignation is another non-productive response. A third is to act in a hostile way, even if you don't say anything. You might refuse to talk to your spouse, for example.

Gaining control over symptoms can reduce frustration and uncertainty. For example, pacing strategies, such as taking regular rests bring greater stability, thus reducing the swings between high symptoms and times of remission, and offering some control over irritability. Resting ahead of an event can make it more likely you can attend. A health log can enable you to see patterns in your symptoms, showing you what makes your symptoms worse. Also, feeling understood can reduce frustration. For ideas on building support, see the section on relationships.

Guilt

Looking back, you may blame yourself for becoming sick. You may scan your past for mistakes you made that resulted in your becoming ill. You might tell yourself things like "If only I had taken better care of myself," "If only I managed stress better" or "If only I had paid better attention to my body." The truth is that no one yet knows the cause of either CFS or fibromyalgia. It is likely that factors over which we have no control, such as genetic susceptibility, will be found to play a major role in both.

We live in a society that sometimes blames people for becoming sick. There is a common idea that if we eat right, exercise and have the right thoughts, we will avoid illness. But the truth is that we are vulnerable, with no control over our genes and subject to many forces we don't understand. Don't buy in to the idea that you wanted to be sick to teach yourself something. Such thoughts only compound the suffering of chronic illness.

You may also feel guilty if you are unable to work or do as much at home as in the past. Living in a society that emphasizes productivity, guilt about doing less than before is common. It is appropriate to look at your situation in a realistic way. If you live with others, your illness probably has caused a redistribution of responsibilities in your family. But it is also helpful to remember that you are not sick by choice and illness has imposed real limits on what you can do.

Guilt can be helpful if it motivates you to take better care of yourself from here forward, but it can be a trap if you see your illness as a personal failure. Whatever happened before, you can exercise control only from the present forward, using such strategies as getting adequate rest, exercising, taking medications to alleviate symptoms, relaxing to reduce stress, developing supportive relationships, accepting a reasonable load of responsibilities (but not more), keeping pleasure in your life, and developing new interests.

Sadness and Depression

Depression and feelings of sadness are common in chronic illness. They are natural responses to loss, uncertainty, limits and the discomfort of symptoms. Depression is a response that lessens further stress or trauma by shutting down, allowing time to process what has already occurred. Depression may also be triggered by a long period of suffering before receiving a diagnosis. Years of inappropriate or insensitive treatment may engender a sense of hopelessness.

Depression usually eases over time. If it lasts, you will have a sense of despair and inertia. Several strategies may be helpful. First, using self-help techniques, such as those discussed in previous chapters, can help you move forward, refuting the belief that all is hopeless. Second, you can work to reframe your thoughts so that they are more realistic and hopeful. (For a three-step process for changing your thinking, see Chapter 31.) Third, since a considerable number of CFS and fibromyalgia patients suffer from clinical depression, you may be helped by professional guidance and medications.

Acceptance

Working through loss is often takes several years. The end point is acceptance, the recognition that life has changed, perhaps permanently and certainly for an extended period of time. Acceptance means letting go of your past life and also of the future as you had envisioned it. And it means saying good-bye to the person you used to be.

Acceptance also includes a realization of the need to live differently than before and a willingness to build a new life. This attitude was summarized by recovered CFS patient Dean Anderson, who said that a certain kind of acceptance was the key to his recovery. He described it not as resignation, but rather "an acceptance of the reality of the illness and of the need to lead a different kind of life, perhaps for the rest of my life." To him, acceptance also means finding ways "to be productive and [to] find fulfillment under unfamiliar and difficult circumstances."

Fibromyalgia patient Joan Buchman outlined a similar process of change in her article "How I Created a Good Life with Fibromyalgia." She wrote that while she did not choose to have fibromyalgia, she did have a choice about how to live with it. She reduced her symptoms through making lifestyle changes and developed a fulfilling life by "focusing on my many blessings."

CFS patient and writer Floyd Skloot describes his journey to acceptance in his memoir *In the Shadow of Memory*. He writes that, after a struggle, he concluded that "since I cannot escape my body and the limits it has imposed on me, I must learn to be at home in it." He says that, over time, he recognized "possibilities for transformation." He found inspiration in Robert Frost's description of acceptance: "Take what is given, and make it over your own way." Skloot concludes that, even though "I may seem shattered. . . there are many ways in which I am better than ever...I feel reborn, hopeful."

Dean, Joan and Floyd all came to an acceptance of the reality of their illness and the need to lead a different kind of life. They found the key to improvement lay in the combination of accepting the illness and disciplining themselves to live in hope within the limits it imposed by CFS or FM.

Strategies for Moving Through Grief

What can help you move through grief? As described above, developing and using a self-management plan offers one way. For example, pacing increases control, thereby replacing frustration, helplessness and uncertainty with stability and predictability. Here are eight additional strategies for moving through grief.

1. **Structure.** Having daily and weekly routines provides a sense of stability and familiarity, counteracting the feelings of disorientation and uncertainty brought by loss. Routine also offers a distraction from loss. Author Gail Cassidy advises, "Do not make any unnecessary major changes in your life during times of loss, as they can further add to the existing instability and anxiety."

2. **Problem Solving.** Respond to the emotions of chronic illness by problem solving. By adopting self-management strategies, you remedy the circumstances that triggered the emotions.

3. **Stress Avoidance.** Having to adjust to the many changes brought by illness is traumatic. In a situation in which you are already overloaded emotionally, it's best to avoid people and situations that add more stress. Gail Cassidy suggests you "stay away from negative people and situations that trigger negative emotions."

4. **Support.** Seek support from family, friends and others. Other people with CFS and FM can provide understanding and models of successful coping. Professional help can give you perspective on your life and help you accept the changes brought by illness.

5. **Acknowledging Grief Triggers.** Grief reactions are often triggered by particular circumstances, such as anniversaries, or by particular people. If your emotions intensify around the anniversary of your becoming ill or on other special dates, plan something positive for those times. If certain people or situations make you feel anxious and uncomfortable, consider limiting your exposure to them.

6. **Acknowledging Loss.** Some people report they found it useful to make a public declaration of loss. One person in our program wrote a Christmas letter to friends to explain why they hadn't heard from him. He wrote, "I am sobered by

the realization that it is highly unlikely that I will return to the level of functioning that I had before becoming ill and so probably will have to adjust to living a life with greater limits than before." He reports writing the letter helped him accept his limits and, paradoxically, increased his resolve to improve.

7. **Recognizing Grief as Cyclic and Long-Term.** You may experience grief repeatedly as you move through the stages of life. For example, you may experience grief if you remain single while friends get married, you remain childless while others become parents, you are not able to be the parent you hoped to be or you can't have the career you trained for.

8. **Addressing Self-Pity.** Almost everyone with chronic illness occasionally feels sorry for themselves. It's not surprising that we would sometimes feel overwhelmed by emotions, given the losses and stresses we experience. Here are four ways to fight back.

   1. *Recognize self-pity is a part of serious illness*. Just as symptoms wax and wane, so do emotions. Acknowledging that self-pity is happening can take some of its power away. You might say something like "Oh, there's self-pity again" or "I see that I'm feeling sorry for myself today." Also, it can help to say consoling things like "I've felt this way before and it's always blown over, so probably it won't last this time either."

   2. *Rest*. Strong emotions are sometimes triggered by fatigue and other symptoms. In those instances, rest may help alleviate both physical symptoms and emotions.

   3. *Connect with others*. Reach out via phone, email or in-person. Sometimes just being in touch can change a mood. At other times it helps to have your mood acknowledged.

   4. *Help others*. Shift your attention off yourself onto what you can do for your family, friends or others in your life.

References

Cassidy, Gail. "CFIDS, Change and Loss," *CFIDS Chronicle* 15(Winter, 2002): 20-21.

CFIDS and Fibromyalgia Self-Help website: *www.cfidsselfhelp.org*. See the Success Stories archive of the Library for the articles by Dean Anderson and Joan Buchman.

Kubler-Ross, Elisabeth. *On Death and Dying*. New York: Macmillan, 1969.

Skloot, Floyd. *In the Shadow of Memory*. Lincoln: University of Nebraska Press, 2003.

27. Creating a New Life

Long-term illness brings pain, suffering and loss, but it also provides an opportunity to reevaluate life and recast it in a new way. Many people in our program have said that, even though they would not have chosen to have CFS or FM, they have learned valuable lessons from it. They believe it is possible to live a rewarding life with long-term illness, even though it is a different kind of life than the one they had before or the one they planned. Some even say they have a better life now than before CFS or FM.

Writing in an article titled "What Recovery Means to Me," JoWynn Johns describes how she recognized and responded to the challenge to build a new life when she says, "Gradually, I came to accept the idea that perhaps I never could go back to my old life." She let go of her goal of recovery, replacing it with the idea of restoring quality of life through building a different kind of life than she had before CFS. "By giving up the need to have what I used to have, by giving up the idea of recovery as return to a past way of living, I have created a good life."

Usually this shift occurs gradually, but sometimes a single experience brings home the finality of loss. A fibromyalgia patient in our program reported that one day she was talking to a friend about her active life before becoming ill and how she had to accept that she couldn't be as active as she used to be. She described her life before illness as including hiking, rock climbing, caving, cross-country skiing, backpacking, orienteering and snow camping. The friend responded by saying, "Yes, that was another life." The patient said her friend's comment was "like someone switching on a light in my brain. Intellectually, I had accepted the loss and I had grieved, but I felt that something was incomplete - suddenly 'that was another life' gave me a file in which to put the old life."

Here are some strategies used by people in our program to build a new life:

Focus on Gains & Improvement

People in our program have echoed JoWynn's sentiments, finding their own ways to give positive meaning to their new lives. One approach is to focus on gains that have occurred because of being ill. Some people in our program say they prefer the person they are today to the one before their illness. One says, "Even though I grieve the loss of self, the new me is a kinder, gentler and more caring person." Another comments, "I actually like the new me better than the old me. I'm much more pleasant to be around and generally more content with life."

Others say that in some respects they have a better life today than before they were ill, with the ability to focus on what is important and more time for relationships. One person wrote, "In many respects, my life now is better than it was before I got sick. I know what my priorities are. I'm not as stressed as I was….I'm almost thankful for having fibromyalgia (and the other related things) because the positives far out weigh the negatives!"

Develop New Interests

A powerful antidote to loss is to develop new interests and, from that, a sense of purpose and meaning. Some people with CFS and FM have taken the opportunity to return to art, crafts or other hobbies that had languished when they were busy with career and family. Taking advantage of newly available time, they start new activities or resume projects they had put aside during their earlier, busier lives.

Others see their illness as a challenge and find a sense of purpose in trying to understand their illness and to expand their area of control. Still others have found meaning in helping others. They may do it through participating in a support group or by offering help informally. Some have started groups or lobbied for better recognition and research funding for CFS and fibromyalgia. Whatever they chose, they found new ways to bring meaning to their life.

One way to bring meaning is to reframe your life in a realistic, yet positive, way. For example, a woman in our program wrote, "I am not the person I was, and I probably won't have the kind of life I thought I would. But whether or not I recover, I try to bring as much meaning as possible to my life now and to value the core qualities in myself that have not changed. I try to remind myself that I still make a difference to other people, and I can still contribute to their lives."

Adjust Goals to Abilities

Focus on those things you can do, rather than on those you can't, and congratulate yourself on your accomplishments. This is sometimes called adjusting expectations to a "new normal" and applies to all family members, not just the person who is ill.

An example is Patti Schmidt's article "Coming to Terms with a Life I Didn't Plan," which describes how she reoriented her life after coming down with CFS. She writes that, after acknowledging that her illness had changed her life irrevocably, she was left with the question: Now what? She made some changes in thinking to accept that there were some things that had been important that she would have to let go of, but she also recognized that she still had what was important to her: her family and the ability to contribute something to others. She decided to focus on those things she could do, rather than on those she couldn't, adjusting her goals to her abilities.

Practice Gratitude

Some people with CFS or FM find it helpful to look at their illness through the lens of gratitude, focusing on their blessings and seeing their illness as a gift. Reflecting on the benefits of keeping a gratitude journal, Joan Buchman wrote that during the time she kept the journal she learned "to treasure what I have right now." Through the journal, she recognized that before becoming ill, "I was not on a track for happiness and peace. Because of FMS, I have had the opportunity to find out what is really important for me to live a fulfilling and meaningful life."

For her, gratitude does not mean that she always looks at the bright side or denies pain and suffering. Rather, for her, gratitude is "appreciating what you have and making the most from it. It's about finding out that you have more power over your life than you previously imagined." (See her article "The Healing Power of Gratitude." Another article, "Counting Your Blessings: How Gratitude Improves Your Health," summarizes scientific research on gratitude.)

Nourish Yourself

Between what you feel you have to do and the suffering imposed by illness, it is easy to let positive things slip out of your life. But we all deserve pleasure and enjoyment. If you have things to look forward to, you help yourself in an important way. The enjoyment of positive experiences reduces stress, replacing it with pleasure and building a positive sense of self-esteem.

Enjoyable experiences may include the physical pleasure that comes from exercise, laughing, taking a bath, listening to or playing music or from intimacy. Or it may be the enjoyment and satisfaction from keeping a garden, painting a picture or completing a crafts project. Or it may be the mental pleasure that comes from enjoying the beauty of nature or from reading a book or the spiritual satisfaction of meditation or prayer.

One person found that solitude had opened a new avenue to appreciation of the arts. She said, "I respond more wholeheartedly to familiar and new literature; to the pictures, wood carvings, and pottery in my room; to the prints, photographs, reproductions of paintings, and needle art I study in books and journals; to music...Experiencing these works alone, without distraction, I find they touch me more deeply, transforming my way of seeing and inspiring my imagination."

Find Positive Models

People in our program report that their adjustment was improved after they met people with CFS and FM who had made positive adjustments to life with long-term illness. Such people provide inspiration and practical ideas for successful adaptation. Also, comparing yourself to other people with CFS and FM is more appropriate than comparisons with healthy people.

Educate Others

Building a new life is difficult if family and friends have outdated and unrealistic expectations of your abilities. Educating them about your illness and limitations is one foundation for positive adaptation. As described in the articles in the Family and Friends archive on our website, all members of the family have to accept a "new normal."

References

CFIDS and Fibromyalgia Self-Help website: *www.cfidsselfhelp.org*. See the Success Stories archive in the Library for the articles by JoWynn Johns, Patti Schmidt and Joan Buchman. See the Coping Strategies archive for the article about research on gratitude.

PART 7

Learn Self-Management Skills

28. Becoming a Self-Manager

With long-term conditions like CFS and fibromyalgia, you have a different role from the one you have with acute illnesses. With short-term illnesses, you often can rely on a doctor to provide a solution or the illness resolves itself. But there is no medical cure so far for either CFS or fibromyalgia. Conditions that can't be cured need to be managed.

A manager is someone who is responsible for making decisions. You are the expert on your condition. You know your situation better than anyone else and you may know more about CFS or fibromyalgia than your doctor. You are the day-to-day manager of your condition. Your decisions and how you lead your life will have a big effect on your symptoms and quality of life.

Self-management involves using a set of skills. Here are six we find particularly useful. (Two of them are discussed in more detail in the next two chapters.)

Educating Yourself

One of your tasks as a self-manager is to gather information about Chronic Fatigue Syndrome and fibromyalgia, learning as much as you can about your condition and the treatment and lifestyle options available to you. Some commonly used sources include patient organizations such as the CFIDS Association of America and the National Fibromyalgia Association; the Internet; support groups; and books and newsletters.

Sorting through all the information can seem overwhelming. Here are two ideas for making that task manageable. First, ask whether the claims you hear are credible. Some people prey on the desperation of patients, so be skeptical of those who promise recovery, particularly if those promises come with a big price tag. Most reliable authorities believe that so far no cure has been developed for either condition. Be willing to experiment, but ask what risks are associated with a treatment and whether the likely gains are consistent with the cost. Second, view education as an ongoing task, but put limits on your efforts. New developments occur from time to time, but breakthroughs are rare. After an initial intense period of educating yourself, you can probably keep up with new ideas by reading to one or two newsletters or magazines. (For some ideas on newsletters, organizations, Internet sites and books, see the article "Educate Yourself" on our website.)

Achieving Goals

Another skill of the self-manager is the ability to set goals and to achieve them. The strategy we use in our program to attain goals is target setting, which involves translating a goal into a series of small, realistic steps or targets. As we use the term, a target is a set of specific actions that you can realistically expect to complete in the near future, typically one week. A target has two characteristics. It is both specific (concrete and measurable) and realistic (doable). The next chapter contains step-by-step instructions for setting targets.

Learning about Yourself: Self-Observation

You are an important source of information about your condition, perhaps the most important one. Using self-observation, you can learn what intensifies your symptoms and what helps you to feel better, and then use that knowledge to improve your quality of life by doing less of those things that make you worse and more of those that help.

Your ability to learn from self-observation can be enhanced greatly by keeping records. Keeping a health diary or log can reveal patterns and show you the links between your actions and your symptoms. Such record keeping should not require more than a few minutes a day. For much more on logging, including sample logs, see Chapter 30.

Experimentation

Finding what works through trial and error is another key skill for successful self-management. Since there are no consistently effective medications for treating CFS or FM, you will probably have to experiment to discover what drugs help you. Experimentation applies to lifestyle change as well. For example, you can use trial and error to determine how much exercise you can tolerate, how far you can drive or how long you can work on the computer.

As mentioned earlier, a woman with a severe case of CFS added several productive hours to her day by trying a different pattern of rest. Instead of taking two rests of three hours each, which had been her practice before taking our class, she tried taking short rests every hour or two. Using this different rest schedule, she cut her total rest time in half, from six hours to three, without increasing her symptoms.

Other people have increased the amount and quality of work they do by being sensitive to time of day. One person found her best time of day for mental activity was in the afternoon. If she studied then, she could read for twice as long as in the morning, with a higher level of understanding.

Reframing Experience

Living successfully with CFS or FM requires not only changing what we do but also what we think, so another skill is making mental adjustments. For example, if you feel guilty with how little you can do now in comparison to your activity level when you were healthy, you may need to adjust your expectations. One person in our program reported that a counselor had helped her to "stop being so hard on myself and accept that I was not pathetic, useless and weak, but was doing a lot to cope with my illness and actually living a pretty worthwhile life in spite of my difficulties."

A related mental adjustment is to change our self-talk or inner dialogue. If you have a tendency to interpret your experience negatively, you can retrain yourself to speak supportively and realistically to yourself when you are depressed or in a flare. You can also change your overall mental climate by noticing what is going right and by congratulating yourself on your accomplishments. Having a positive focus doesn't mean denying problems or ignoring symptoms, but involves taking heart in progress and seeing successes as signs that improvement is possible. For more on this topic, see Chapter 31 and the articles "Optimism, Hope and Control" and "Counting Your Blessings: How Gratitude Improves Your Health" on our website.

Problem Solving

Problem solving is the master skill. It gives you a structured way to respond to issues that arise in your life. You can think of it as a four-step process.

1) Select a Problem

The starting point is to identify a problem that is important to you and that you feel ready or compelled to work on now. It will usually be something that interferes with your life, makes your life much more difficult or prevents you from doing something that is important to you. Here are two examples.

- For years before becoming ill, you hosted your family's holiday celebration. You decorated your house and cooked the meal. Even though you are now ill and too much activity triggers a flare up of your symptoms, you feel pressured to entertain your family in the same way as before. You would like to find a way to celebrate the holidays that doesn't trigger a relapse.

- Doing your weekly laundry and other household chores tires you out so much that you need more rest than usual for two days afterwards. You hate a messy house and not having clean clothes, but you can't see how to do your chores, given your limited energy

2) List and Evaluate Possible Solutions

The second step is to consider solutions. Begin by listing as many possibilities as you can imagine. Often, problems have multiple causes, so a combination of solutions may be appropriate. After you have a list, consider advantages and disadvantages of each option, and then rank them, giving the highest place to the solution you believe is most likely to work. Here's one way the second step might unfold in our examples.

Holiday Celebration: Solutions to your holiday dilemma include: hosting the celebration, but having others bring the food; rotating the celebration among other relatives; and hosting the holiday meal in a restaurant.

Each solution requires that you and your family examine and modify how the work of holiday celebrations is handled. A solution will probably involve family conversations in which you may need to be assertive about your limits and your need for help. There are psychological adjustments as well. Giving up your role as host for the holidays is just one part of a broader experience of loss.

Household Chores: You are not able to do your household chores in the way you used to. One possible solution is to spread the chores out over several days rather than doing everything in one day. Or you might still do all your chores in one day, but in small chunks, taking frequent rest breaks.

Another possible solution is to clean less frequently. (One person with FM wrote she now views dust as something that "protects my furniture.") As with some of the solutions for holiday celebrations, this involves changing your ideas of what is appropriate. Two other solutions involve getting help from others. You might ask family members to share in the work. For example, children could clean their own rooms and do their own laundry. Or you could hire a cleaning service.

A final possibility is to move to a smaller home. If you saw housecleaning as one example of how household responsibilities in general had become too great, you might consider simplifying your life by moving to a home that is easier to maintain. People in our groups have used all of these strategies.

3) Experiment with Solutions

The third step is to try various solutions and evaluate the results. Probably some potential remedies won't work, but others may. Here's one way the third step could turn out in our examples.

Holiday Celebration: You talk to your husband and children about a new division of labor for the holidays. You agree to have a less ambitious event this year. Your extended family, however, is unsympathetic. They have never believed you are really sick. You and your husband agree to host the family celebration for at least one more year. He and your children agree to share cooking responsibilities. You conclude that it may take several years to settle into a new holiday routine that all family members will accept. You also decide that some members of your extended family may never accept your limits. You join a support group and find it helpful to talk to other people with fibromyalgia about accepting the loss of your old role in the family.

Household Chores: After talking with friends from a support group, you decide to try a combination of strategies. You ask your children to clean their own rooms and wash their own laundry. Also, you decide you will reduce the amount of housecleaning you do, cleaning less thoroughly and having your house cleaned twice a year by professionals. At the suggestion of another patient, you decide to keep a journal to explore your thoughts and feelings about the loss of your ability to "keep up."

4) Evaluate Results

Assess the results of your experiments. It's possible that some of your experiments will be successful, but that others may not. If you don't have a complete success, you may have a partial solution. Your final solution may be a combination of several approaches. It may be helpful to look at your efforts as a series of experiments. With that view, you can more easily accept disappointments and move on to another attempt. In some cases, a problem may not be solvable or not solvable at the present time.

Summary

There are a number of principles to keep in mind while using problem solving.

- **Explore a variety of potential solutions**. There are often several ways a problem can be solved. Looking at your situation from a number of perspectives can help you recognize different approaches. Some problems are solved by a combination of strategies.

- **Ask what resources are available**. In many cases, you will be able to solve your problems yourself by brainstorming possible solutions and trying one or more of them. But, you may sometimes want to get help, either in trying to understand your problem or in solving it.

- **Practice assertiveness**. Your illness will require changes in your role and in those of other members of your family. Tasks like grocery shopping and hosting the family holiday celebration may need to be renegotiated. You have to adjust to the loss of roles, while others often must take on new responsibilities.

- **Make mental and emotional adjustments**. Having a serious illness requires that you adopt new expectations for yourself based on having new, more restrictive limits. You will probably have to reduce your activity level and also make psychological adjustments, accepting that the person you were before your illness has been replaced with a new, more limited person.

References

CFIDS and Fibromyalgia Self-Help website: *www.cfidsselfhelp.org*. The article on educating yourself is in the series "Eight Steps to a Better Life." The articles on optimism and gratitude are in the Coping Strategies section of the Library.

29. *Goals and Targets*

One skill of the self-manager is the ability to achieve goals. The technique we use in our program for attaining goals is *target setting,* which involves translating a goal into a series of small, realistic steps or targets. (Other self-help programs use this technique, but they may call it by different names, such as *contracting* or making an *action plan*.)

Target setting involves three steps: making a realistic short-term plan, carrying it out, and evaluating the results.

Make a Plan

A target has two characteristics: it is specific and realistic. *Specific* means that a target is concrete and measurable. For example, instead of saying "I want to get more rest," you say "I will rest 15 minutes in the late morning on four days in the next week." The plan you create should answer the following questions:

- **What specifically will you do?** For example, will you rest, phone a friend or take a series of walks?

- **How much?** If your target is to rest, will you rest for 15 minutes, an hour or some other length of time?

- **When?** Will you rest in the morning, afternoon, evening or some combination?

- **How often?** How many days a week will you do your target? You may want to do something daily, but you're more likely to succeed if you allow yourself some "breathing room" by aiming to do something several times a week rather than every day.

To test whether your target is *realistic*, ask your self how confident you are that you can complete your target as stated. Answer by giving a number between 0 and

10, where 0 means "not confident at all" and 10 means "totally confident." Your confidence level is your estimation of how sure you are that you can complete the target *in its entirety*, not a measure of how much of the target you will complete.

If the answer is 8 or higher, you have a good chance to succeed. If your confidence level is lower than 8, restate your goal in less ambitious terms. For example, you can increase your chances of success if you reduce the number of times per week that you rest from everyday to four or five days. Or, for an exercise target, reduce the length of time you exercise from 15 minutes to ten minutes.

An alternative response if your confidence is low is to ask what might stop you from achieving your goal. For example, if you want to exercise outside, bad weather might make that difficult. If you can identify potential problems, you may be able to come up with solutions. Alternative ways to exercise in bad weather might be to walk in a mall or use an exercise video at home. Once you have considered alternatives, you can ask yourself if your confidence level has changed. Stop this process once your answer is 8 or higher, meaning that you are quite confident that you can complete the whole target as stated.

You are more likely to succeed if you keep a few other ideas in mind. First, your target should be something that *you* want to do, not something that others want or something that you think you "should" do. Second, start by setting a one target per week. This gives you a chance to learn how to use targeting. It takes a while to develop a new skill. The purpose of target setting is to help you have an experience of taking an active role in managing your illness. Third, accept yourself as you are and begin by aiming to make a small change. If you do, you are likely to succeed and your success will build on itself, boosting your self-confidence.

Implement

After you have formulated your plan, write it down on the Target form. (You can find a blank target form at the end of this chapter. Also, there is a printable version of this and all the other forms in this book on our website: *www.cfidsselfhelp.org*. Go to the Library section and click on Logs, Forms & Worksheets.)

Write your target and confidence level in the section labeled "My Target." Putting your intention in writing helps strengthen your commitment. Other ways to make it more likely that you will follow through include telling other people about your plan and posting your target in a place where you are likely to see it frequently, such as on the refrigerator.

As the week unfolds, track your efforts by filling out the second section of the form, "Results." Use this space to write down what you've done and any problems that have arisen. Putting your experience in writing is a good way to hold yourself accountable and thereby increase your chances for success.

Evaluate

At the end of a week, evaluate your results by asking how successful you were in meeting your target. The two most common problems people experience in target setting are not being specific and being too ambitious. The solution to the first is to ask whether your target answers the four questions of what, how much, when and how often. The solution to the second is to ask whether your confidence level is at least 8 on a scale of 0 to 10.

Even if your target is well stated and seems realistic, you may still experience problems. Perhaps the unpredictability of your illness prevents you from completing the target as planned. Or, you may decide that your target is not realistic at this time. But, whatever the results, you can learn from your efforts. To help you gain something positive regardless of the outcome, fill out the "Lessons" section of the form.

It can be helpful to view your target setting as a series of experiments. If you meet your target, you have a successful experiment and can gain some control over your illness. If the results are different from your expectations, you can learn something useful about your illness by reflecting on your experience.

Sample Targets

You can make a target in practically any area of life. Here are some real examples used by people in our program.

Rest for 20 minutes each: late morning and mid-afternoon
Taking scheduled rests is one of the most common targets used by people in our groups. For more on rest, see the chapter on pacing strategies.

Go to bed by 10 pm
The person who set this target wanted to re-establish a more normal routine after staying up later and later.

Get off computer after 30 minutes
You can set a target not to do something or to set a limit on how much you do.

Find a nanny to help with childcare
Both the woman who set this target and her daughter have CFS. The mother thought that by having someone come in several times a week, her daughter would have more companionship and the mother could have some free time.

Talk to my wife about our relationship

The man who set this target was worried about the extra responsibilities imposed on his wife by his illness and wondered how they could handle all the uncertainty created by his CFS. Making this commitment to his class motivated him to have a long-postponed conversation.

Read a book for pleasure

This target was used by a person who thought that the demands of family and illness had squeezed all the pleasure out of her life. It may seem paradoxical to schedule pleasure, but it worked.

One Person's Experience

Let's look at the experience one person in our program had with her first target. This woman found the idea of scheduled rest periods appealing as a way to reduce her symptoms. Using the idea of rest as lying down with her eyes closed in a quiet place, she set a target of resting 15 minutes every afternoon for a week. This target answered the four questions. It defined what she was going to do (*rest*), how much (*15 minutes*), when (*afternoon*), and how often (*daily*).

Next she asked herself how confident she was that she could complete the target as stated. Her answer was 6. She realized that she wasn't confident she could do something every day, so she changed her target to aim for four days rather than every day. With this less ambitious goal, she rated her confidence at 8. She wrote her target as:

What	Rest
How much	15 minutes
When	Mid-afternoon
How often	Four days in the next week
Confidence	8

She began the week successfully, resting for 15 minutes on Monday afternoon. She got up feeling more energetic and less brain fogged. On Tuesday, she lay down as scheduled but got up after a few minutes when the phone rang. The call was from a friend and they talked for half an hour. When the call ended, she gave up on the idea of rest for that day. On Wednesday, she unplugged the phone before lying down. A call came in during her rest, but she let the answering machine take it. She got up feeling refreshed by the rest.

On Thursday, she did some errands in the mid-afternoon and didn't attempt a nap. She rested on Friday, but got up feeling worse. She felt preoccupied by a worry about her daughter's progress in school. Her mind was spinning during her rest. As a result, the time lying down didn't feel very restful.

The entries she made in the "Results" section of her target form were as follows:

Mon   Felt better after
Tue   Stopped to answer phone
Wed   Ignored call
Fri   Felt worse after: worried

Lastly, she evaluated her experience with rest. She congratulated herself on nearly meeting her target. She rested 15 minutes for three days, with some rest on a fourth. She concluded that her experience was enough to show her the value of resting. She had more energy after at least some of the rests, gaining a sense that rest might offer a way to control her illness.

In thinking about the worry that had interfered with her rest on Friday, she remembered hearing about relaxation techniques and asked herself whether she might practice them while resting. She thought that doing so might help her rest her mind as well as her body, giving her a way to reduce her worry. In the "Lessons" section of her target form, she wrote:

Resting can be helpful. Want to try relaxation as part of rest.

Getting Started

Now it's your turn. Think of a problem that bothers you. Pick just one and commit to making a start today. Then, brainstorm several possible solutions, things that might reduce or solve your problem. After reviewing them, pick one to try in the next week and write down a target that answers the four questions: what, how much, when and how often?

Once you've stated your target, ask yourself how confident you are that you can complete it successfully. Give your confidence a number between 0 (meaning no confidence) and 10 (totally confident). If your confidence is less than 8, restate your goal in less ambitious terms. Once you have a target and feel confident about achieving it, you're ready to go. Give your target a try for a week, and then look at the results. If you meet your target, congratulate yourself. If you don't, ask yourself what lessons you can learn from the experience.

My Target

What _____

How Much _____

When _____

How Often _____

Confidence Level _____
(0 = no confidence; 10=totally confident)

Results

Day   Comments

1

2

3

4

5

Lessons

What I Learned _____

_____

_____

30. Logs, Worksheets and Rules

Another skill of the self-manager is self-observation. Through becoming aware of the effects of your activity level, your thoughts and your feelings, you can learn what intensifies your symptoms and what helps you to feel better. Then, by changing how you live, you can do less of those things that make you worse and more of those that help.

Your ability to learn from self-observation can be enhanced greatly by keeping records. The first section of this chapter describes record keeping using health logs. Taking a few minutes a day to fill out a log can help you uncover links between events in your life and your symptom level. Then you can use worksheets and other resources described in the second part of the chapter to translate the insights from your logging into plans, rules and personal guidelines.

Keeping a Health Log

A health log can help you in at least four ways. You can use records to:

- Control symptoms
- Motivate yourself
- Get a reality check
- Explain and document your illness

Controlling Symptoms

If you are like most people with CFS and fibromyalgia, your symptoms fluctuate, both within a day and from one day to the next. When these fluctuations seem random, they can contribute to a sense of frustration and helplessness. A health log offers a way to understand the fluctuations in your symptoms, a tool for discovering what makes your illness worse and what helps you feel better. This knowledge opens the way to your gaining some control over your symptoms.

For example, records can help you learn how to pace yourself. One person in our program noticed that her symptoms were proportional to her exertion. She used her logs to divide activities into categories of light, moderate and heavy, based on how much energy each activity required and how much it increased her symptoms. Then she used that information to plan her days so that she could alternate light activities with moderate and heavy ones. She reported, "I can do more now and have lower symptoms."

Other people report that record keeping helped them to recognize that many different factors contribute to their symptoms. In addition to physical activity, they may include emotional events, stress, social activity and sensory information. If you are sensitive to sound and/or light, you might limit your socializing to quiet settings with lighting you can tolerate.

Another factor that can affect symptoms is time of day. One woman used record keeping and experimentation to discover that she is much more alert in the afternoon. When she read in the morning, fibro fog set in after 15 minutes to half an hour, but her mental stamina was much better in the afternoon. By studying after lunch, she was able to read for two 30-minute sessions with a 10-minute break and could retain the information. Over time, she increased her total study time to two hours a day. Keeping records showed her that *when* she did something was crucially important.

Records can also show how the effects of activity may be delayed. One person noticed that he felt unusually tired some days in the late afternoon. Through studying his records, he found that these episodes occurred on days when he had exercised earlier in the day. He was surprised at this connection, because he hadn't experienced symptoms while exercising. He experimented with different levels of exercise, eventually finding one that didn't tire him out.

Records can reveal the cumulative effects of activity, showing the importance of looking at periods longer than a day. Some people find that they can maintain a consistent activity level for several days, feeling tired only at the end of the period. Having records helps them think about what level of activity they can sustain.

You can also use your records to understand patterns over even longer periods of time. One person in our program, for example, used his daily logs to understand, and then eliminate, relapses. Reviewing his logs for a year in which he had spent a total of almost two weeks in bed with CFS flares, he found that most of his relapses were associated with either travel or secondary illnesses, such as colds or the flu.

To minimize travel-related setbacks, he decided to limit travel to a few hours' driving distance from home and to take rest breaks while driving. He decided to combat relapses triggered by secondary illnesses by taking extra rest after the symptoms of the secondary illness had ended. In the decade since making those changes, he has experienced no relapses.

Motivating Yourself

Records can also be an important source of motivation and inspiration. Seeing written proof that activity level affects symptoms can provide a stimulus to stick with pacing. Records of progress can provide hope. CFS patient JoWynn Johns, says in her article "Living Within My Envelope," that both factors were important to her. After recognizing that mental exertion and emotional stress provoked her symptoms just as much as physical activities, she concluded that she would need records to remind herself of those causes of her symptoms. And, she writes, "Color coding with hi-liters enables me to see readily how I'm doing during the month. I find this kind of visible feedback motivating."

Getting a Reality Check

Records can also function like a mirror, offering a reality check. One person in our program said, "Logging brings home to me the reality of my illness. Before logging, I didn't realize that most of my time is spent on or below about 35% functionality. This false perception that I was better than I am led me to overdo things, but now I am less ambitious."

Another person uses a visual record keeping system to help her pace herself. She rates each day and records her rating on a calendar using colored dots. Green means a good day. Yellow means caution. Red means stop: intense symptoms, time to go to bed.

A third person reviews her records to see where she might accept more responsibility. "At the end of each week, I look at my activity log and write a short summary at the bottom of the page, commenting on good experiences, symptoms I had that were not my fault, and symptoms I had [that] I could have had some control over."

Explaining Your Illness & Documenting Disability

Lastly, you can use records in discussions with physicians and in substantiating a claim for disability. Health records can document your functional level and show changes over time.

Sample Health Diaries

There are many ways to track your life using written records. Here are two health diaries to get you started. You can use one or both of them or develop your own system.

Symptom Log

The Symptom Log consists of a list of symptoms common to people with CFS and fibromyalgia. (There is a sample log and a blank form at the end of the chapter. Also, blank forms are available on our website: *www.cfidsselfhelp.org*. Go to the Library section and click on Logs, Forms & Worksheets.) To use the log, make entries one or more times a day, using one column for each set of entries.

You can use this log to:

- Define your overall level of symptoms
- Determine which symptoms are most important
- Document daily swings in symptoms
- Recognize interactions among symptoms
- Document changes in symptom levels over time

The example at the end of the chapter shows a Symptom Log completed for a five-day period. The chart shows a symptom cluster consisting of five elements: fatigue, pain, fogginess/memory problems, poor sleep and depression. These symptoms were at moderate to severe levels during at least part of every day. In addition, this person had two days with headaches.

The log indicates that the person's symptoms usually improved during the day and were generally lowest at night. The exceptions were Wednesday and Thursday, when she was more active than usual in the afternoon. The effects of overactivity were delayed, not occurring until the evening.

The person using the log also observed some connections among symptoms. Her main symptoms (fatigue, brain fog, and muscle pain) were lowest in the mornings that followed nights with good sleep. She also saw a connection between depression and her other symptoms. Her depression was lowest when her other symptoms lightened in the morning, and higher when she experienced stronger symptoms.

Activity Log

The Activity Log helps you associate activities with symptom levels. Using the log, you can recognize connections between causes (your activities and the events in your life) and effects (your symptoms). Activities you might want to track include amount and quality of sleep and rest, specific activities (cooking, errands, TV, reading, socializing), exercise, emotions and stress.

You'll find a blank activity log at the end of the chapter. Using it, you can record the number of hours of sleep (entered for the day the sleep ended), daytime rest, key activities and events of the day, symptoms with severity rated from 1 to 10, comments and an overall rating for the day on a scale of 1 to 5. On this scale, 1 is a very poor day, 3 is an average day and 5 a very good day.

To give you an idea of how to use the form, there is a sample Activity Log at the end of the chapter. The person who filled it out was interested in finding patterns in her symptoms and associating the patterns with events in her life. Before starting her record keeping, she noticed an improvement in her symptoms due to two changes she made. She had more stamina after starting two half-hour pre-emptive rests each day. Also, she reduced her brain fog and became more productive in her half-time job after changing her work schedule from mornings, when her symptoms are usually worse, to afternoons, a better time of day for her.

Even after making these changes, she had a higher level of symptoms than she wanted, so was motivated to start logging to identify some reasons why. She decided to make entries in her log three times a day. She planned to enter the number of hours she slept at night as soon as she woke up. She also expected to write entries just before going to work and at bedtime.

She rated Monday as average (3). During the morning, she had mild pain and fatigue, plus a small amount of brain fog. She experienced no symptoms in the afternoon, her best time of day. In the evening, she felt moderate brain fog during dinner in a noisy restaurant and had trouble getting to sleep.

On Tuesday, she had a higher level of symptoms in the morning, plus symptoms in the afternoon. For this reason, she rated the day as below average. She asked herself why she had higher than usual symptoms. There was no obvious cause on Tuesday for the flare. Her activity level was similar to that on an average day. But her activity level on Monday had been higher than normal. In addition to her time at work, she had done shopping and cooking in the morning, and had gone out in the evening. Also, she had skipped her rest after sleeping poorly on Sunday night. Her experience was probably an example of how the effects of events can be delayed. Record keeping can help make delayed reactions more evident.

Because her symptoms were even more intense on Wednesday, she rated that day as much below average. She rested in the morning, which helped reduce her symptoms somewhat, but she left work early. She was probably feeling the cumulative effects of several days' activity.

On Thursday, she felt a little better when she got up and spent much of the morning resting before going to work. That rest, in combination with all the rest the previous day, seemed to help her back to an average level of symptoms overall. She noted that fibro fog set in after she had been on the computer for 45 minutes. This experience indicates that exceeding limits on mental activity can lead to symptoms.

She forgot to note her activities on Friday morning, but rated the day as better than usual because of having low symptoms in the morning and none in the afternoon or evening. She slipped back to below average on Saturday after spending part of the afternoon doing errands and an hour gardening. The combination resulted in her standing for a total of three hours, much beyond her one-hour limit. She decided to keep a movie date with a friend for the evening, even though her symptoms were moderate.

Her symptoms were only a little above average on Sunday morning, but she was able to eliminate them by resting for several hours. The rest of the day was symptom-free, except for an hour in the evening, when she experienced moderate brain fog following a phone conversation with her sister. Her sister had called to announce that she was pregnant. The person was excited by the news, then remembered that emotional events, whether good or bad, often trigger brain fog.

Guidelines for Logging

If you are interested in using health logs, you might keep in mind the following two guidelines. Make your log:

1. **Easy to Use.** If your diary is easy to use, you are more likely to fill it out. A common rule of thumb is that a log should take only a few minutes a day to fill out.

2. **Meaningful to You.** Use logging to help you answer questions that are important to you, not because you think you should or to please others. Whether you use an existing form or develop your own system, make sure the records fit your situation.

Record on a daily basis and set aside time regularly to review your logs. Plan to spend some time on a regular basis (for example, once every week or two) going over what you have written to look for patterns and connections. If possible, ask someone to go over them with you.

Planning Forms & Personal Rules

Taking what you have learned from your logging, you can create a set of individualized guides for better living. The Daily and Weekly Schedule worksheets, described in Chapter 10, give you a way to translate your understanding of your capabilities and limits into daily and weekly routines. The Relapse Worksheet, described in Chapter 13, is a way to summarize your learning about what causes your relapses and how to minimize them.

Another type of guide used by people in our program is personalized rules for living well with CFS and FM. These can take three forms. First, you might state a few rules crucial to controlling symptoms. An example is the person mentioned earlier who has three rules for herself: no more than three trips outside the house per week, no driving beyond 12 miles from home, and no phone conversations longer than 20 minutes.

Second, you may set rules covering many circumstances. For example, after you have defined your limits, you can establish rules for how long you stay on the computer, how long you talk on the phone, how much exercise you do, how far you drive, when you go to bed at night and get up in the morning, when you rest during the day, how long you spend in social situations and so on.

Third, you might write down your strategies for symptom management. For example, for managing fatigue, people in our program often mention taking daily rests, getting enough sleep, limiting the number of times they leave the house each week, breaking up tasks into small chunks and limiting the time spent standing up. For managing pain, common strategies include pain medications, exercise, adequate sleep, daily rests, massage and heat and/or cold.

A related idea is, to quote the title of an article on our website, to develop a set of "Personal Guidelines for Managing Chronic Illness." The idea with this approach is to have a few principles to guide your life with chronic illness and to be a reference in times of confusion. Here's what I came up with for myself. The words in italics went on a 3 x 5 card for quick reference; I printed the full text on a sheet of paper.

1) Live within my energy envelope

I believe I can reduce symptoms and regain control by living within my limits. For me, this means taking scheduled rests daily, keeping a daily log, returning only gradually to my normal routine after a relapse or illness and avoiding stressful people and situations.

2) Extend the envelope gradually

Recognizing that CFS controls the timetable and extent of my improvement, I will experiment occasionally to expand my activity level, but not more than 5% to 10% at a time. I recognize that not all my experiments will work.

3) When all else fails, go to bed

There are times when the best course is to surrender to the illness. This guideline gives me permission to acknowledge that at times I am powerless over the disease and the smartest course is to give in to it.

4) Accept that I may not recover

I believe I can create the conditions for recovery but can't control whether I recover. Thus, I try to focus on feeling better, which I believe *is* under my control to some degree.

To organize your logs, forms, worksheets and rules, consider using a three ring binder with several dividers. Label the tabs on the dividers in a way that's helpful to you. You might have tabs for worksheets, plus others for your logs, one for your rules and another for a list of your medications. Alternately, you could keep your materials in file folders or organize them in some other way. The important thing is to develop a system that fits your situation.

Resources

Copeland, Mary Ellen. *Winning Against Relapse*. Oakland: New Harbinger, 1999.

Starlanyl, Devin and Mary Ellen Copeland. *Fibromyalgia & Chronic Myofascial Pain: A Survival Manual*. Oakland: New Harbinger, 2001. 2nd ed. (See Chapter 16: Wellness Recovery Action Planning.)

FlyLady website: *www.flylady.com*. (See section titled "Control Journal.")

Symptom Log

Symptoms	Mon am	Mon pm	Mon eve	Tue am	Tue pm	Tue eve	Wed am	Wed pm	Wed eve	Thr am	Thr pm	Thr eve	Fri am	Fri pm	Fri eve
Fatigue	7	6	5	5	4	5	5	4	6	7	5	7	7	5	5
Pain	6	4	3	4	2	2	4	2	4	6	4	3	4	2	2
Fogginess/Memory	7	6	5	5	4	5	5	4	6	7	5	7	7	5	5
Poor Sleep	7			4			4			7			5		
Abdominal Pain															
Depression	5	4	4	1	2	4	1	0	3	5	3	5	5	3	3
Dizziness															
Headaches					4	2				5				3	2
Joint Pain															
Light/Sound Sensitivity															
Lymph Node Tenderness															
Numbness/Tingling															
Sore Throat															

Scale:

None	Mild	Moderate	Severe	Very Severe
0	1-3	4-6	7-9	10

Activity Log

Day	Hours Sleep	Hours Rest	Activities and Events	Symptoms & Severity				Comments	Rating
				Pain	Fatig	Fog	Other		
Mon	7.5	0	am Shopping & cooking	3	3	1			3
			pm Work				Agitated (4)	Noisy restaurant	
			eve Dinner Out			4			
Tue	6	1	am Housecleaning	5	4	3			2
			pm Work	3	2	2			
			eve Rest, TV						
Wed	6	3	am Rest	7	6	5			1
			pm Work	5	4	4	Headache (4)	left early	
			eve Rest, Phone, TV	4	3				
Thr	8	2	am Rest	3	3	1			3
			pm Work					Fog after 45 min on net	
			eve TV, Internet, TV			4			
Fri	8.5	1	am	3	3	1			4
			pm Work						
			eve TV, Phone						
Sat	8	2	am Read & rest	3	3	3			2
			pm Errands & garden	6	5	3			
			eve Movie	5	4	4			
Sun	6	3	am Rest	4	3	3			3
			pm Shopping					Better after rest	
			eve TV, phone			4		Sister pregnant	

Symptom Log

Symptoms	Mon am	Mon pm	Mon eve	Tue am	Tue pm	Tue eve	Wed am	Wed pm	Wed eve	Thr am	Thr pm	Thr eve	Fri am	Fri pm	Fri eve
Fatigue															
Pain															
Fogginess/Memory															
Poor Sleep															
Abdominal Pain															
Depression															
Dizziness															
Headaches															
Joint Pain															
Light/Sound Sensitivity															
Lymph Node Tenderness															
Numbness/Tingling															
Sore Throat															

Scale: None 0   Mild 1-3   Moderate 4-6   Severe 7-9   Very Severe 10

Activity Log

Day	Hours Sleep	Hours Rest	Activities and Events	Symptoms & Severity				Comments	Rating
				Pain	Fatig	Fog	Other		
Mon									
Tue									
Wed									
Thr									
Fri									
Sat									
Sun									

31. New Thoughts and New Habits

Living well with CFS or fibromyalgia requires changing both what we think and what we do. This chapter deals with both. We'll discuss mental adjustments first, then how to change habitual behaviors.

We've seen many examples of mental adjustments throughout the book. One came up in the discussion of pacing. In order to live within our limits, we have to adjust our expectations to fit our current abilities. We also saw that changing our inner dialogue is one way to reduce pain, because dwelling on negative thoughts increases the experience of pain. Similarly, our subjective experience of pain is increased by emotions such as depression and anxiety that are associated with negative thoughts, so managing our feelings by changing our thoughts offers one way to control pain. Also, we can reduce the suffering experienced during relapses by saying comforting things to ourselves.

Mental adjustments are important for controlling stress as well, because thoughts can be a source of stress. For example, if you experience stress because you think that as a "good wife" or "good mother" you should keep your house as you did before becoming ill or should contribute more in other ways, you can reduce your stress by changing your expectations to fit your new limits.

Three-Step Approach

The three-step approach you'll learn now will show you how to change your thoughts so they help you rather than increase your suffering. Having realistic ideas about your situation can help you pace and will reduce pain, stress and the suffering of relapses.

We will focus on our inner dialogue or self-talk. Self-talk is a habitual way of responding to experience, often an internal critic who can be very pessimistic. For example, if you experience a relapse, your inner voice might say something like, "You'll never get any better. Every time you try something, you fail."

Sometimes the internal voice is misleading in a positive direction, if it says things like "This new treatment will cure me for sure."

Your self-talk can have a big effect on your mood and your self-esteem. Unnecessarily negative thoughts make you feel anxious, sad and hopeless. These feelings, in turn, make it difficult to act constructively. Preoccupation with suffering may even intensify symptoms and trigger more negative thinking. The cycle can be very demoralizing, making it difficult to motivate yourself. Similarly, it can be demoralizing to experience repeated cycles of unrealistic hope for recovery followed by disappointment.

Recognizing Automatic Thoughts

The first step to changing your habitual thinking is to recognize it. This is not easy to do because our thoughts are automatic, so deeply ingrained that they seem self-evident. But if you can recognize the thoughts, you gain some distance from them and remove their self-evident character.

The technique I will outline for recognizing and gradually changing automatic thoughts is the Thought Record, which is described in the book *Mind Over Mood* by Dennis Greenberger and Christine Padesky. Using this form offers one way to become aware of automatic thoughts and their effects on your mood and behavior. You can find similar techniques in other books, such as *Learned Optimism* by Martin Seligman or *Feeling Good* by David Burns or learn them from psychologists who specialize in cognitive therapy.

To see how this technique works, imagine a patient who took a walk one day and felt very tired when she got home. Feeling depressed and hopeless, she asked herself what thoughts were going through her mind at that point. They were, "I'll never get better. Every time I try something, it fails." She recorded her experience in the first three columns of the Thought Record (next page). In column 1, she wrote a description of the event. In the second column, she recorded her emotions at the time of the event. And, in the third column, she wrote the thoughts going through her mind when the emotions were strongest.

The purpose of this exercise is to help you gain some distance from your thoughts, to remove their taken-for-granted or self-evident character. Because these thoughts are automatic, they can be hard to recognize and it can take some time to develop this skill. To capture your automatic thoughts, fill out a Thought Record as soon as you can when an upsetting event occurs.

Thought Record #1		
1	2	3
Event	Emotions	Initial Thoughts
Walked 30 min. Very tired after	depressed hopeless	I'll never get better. Every time I try something, it fails.

Evaluating Automatic Thoughts

Once you identify your automatic thoughts by recording them, evaluate them to separate truth from distortions and irrationalities. To help you determine to what extent your automatic thoughts are valid, ask yourself what is the evidence for and against your thoughts. Use column 4 in the Thought Record for evidence in favor of your initial thoughts and column 5 for evidence against.

Thought Record #2				
1	2	3	4	5
Event	Emotions	Initial Thoughts	Pro	Con
Walked 30 min. Very tired after	depressed hopeless	I'll never get better. Every time I try something, it fails.	I have frequent setbacks. Exercise often makes me worse.	Overall, I'm better than a year ago. Many people improve.

The idea is to suspend your belief that the automatic thoughts are true and, instead, look for evidence both pro and con. Writing down the evidence you find helps you gain distance from your thoughts and makes them less self-evident. By stepping back, you can more easily see how your automatic thoughts may ignore facts or select only the worst aspects of a situation.

Your thoughts at moments of strong emotion may seem irrefutable, so it may help to have in mind some questions you can ask yourself in order to find evidence that does not support your thoughts. Among them:

- Do I know of situations in which the thought is not completely true all the time?
- If someone else had this thought, what would I tell them?
- When I felt this way in the past, what did I think that helped me feel better?
- Five years from now, am I likely to view this situation differently?
- Am I blaming myself for something not under my control?

Seeing Alternatives

In the last step, you propose a new understanding of your experience. What you write in column 6 of the Thought Record should be either an alternative interpretation of your experience (if you refuted the thought) or a balanced thought that summarizes the valid points for and against (if the evidence was mixed). In either case, what you write should be consistent with the evidence you recorded in columns 4 and 5. At first, this process may seem artificial and contrived, but it has a point: you are training yourself to use a more balanced and realistic explanatory style. You are learning to replace one habitual interpretation of experience with another.

Reviewing what she had written in columns 4 and 5, our patient decided that the evidence was mixed. She wrote in column 6 a balanced thought that combined the evidence for and the evidence against. "I have frequent relapses and don't know if I will have lasting improvement, but I've made progress and that gives me hope."

Thought Record #3					
1	2	3	4	5	6
Event	Emotions	Initial Thoughts	Pro	Con	Corrected Thoughts
Walked 30 min. Very tired after	depressed hopeless	I'll never get better. Every time I try something, it fails.	I have frequent setbacks. Exercise often makes me worse.	Overall, I'm better than a year ago. Many people improve.	I have frequent relapses and don't know if I will have lasting improvement, but I've made progress and that gives me hope.

Realistic Thinking, Not Positive Thinking

The three-step approach involves changing deeply ingrained habits of thought. The long-term results can be dramatic, but improvement is gradual, and there may be some bumps along the road. Becoming aware of negative thoughts may produce a short-term drop in mood.

The process suggested here does *not* involve replacing negative thoughts with positive, but inaccurate, thoughts. I am not suggesting you adopt something like the motto "every day, in every way, I am getting better and better." Rather, the goal is to learn to see your situation in an accurate, yet hopeful, manner: retraining your habits of thought in a more realistic direction.

The kind of thinking advocated here integrates all evidence, both positive and negative, in a realistic, balanced fashion. Using this way of understanding your experience, you acknowledge the negatives in your life, but praise yourself for your successes. This approach should reduce your stress by helping you feel better, less anxious and sad. And, at the same time, it should help you to deal more effectively with your illness.

Habit Change

Changing habitual thoughts is related to changing habitual behaviors. Let me explain using an example of a person in our program who changed how she handles household tasks. When she was healthy, her attitude was "I work until the task is done." When she got fibromyalgia, she found that approach made her symptoms worse. Over time, she replaced her previous approach with the thought "I stop when tired." The new thought has led to new habits such as taking rest breaks while cleaning or cooking. The new habits have given her a sense of control.

Habit change begins with awareness. For this woman, awareness meant the recognition that, with fibromyalgia in her life, her old attitude toward household tasks led not to a sense of accomplishment, but rather to intensified symptoms and a sense of helplessness. At this stage, the goal is not habit change, but rather awareness of the consequences of continuing old habits.

The second step of habit change is the creation of alternative behavior. In our example, the alternative was to stop when tired. The key to success in this step is to plan a response ahead of time, so that when a situation arises, you can do something different than in the past.

One way to change behavior is to create and use a set of personal rules. Rules describe what you will do in a given situation. For example, you might establish rules for how long to stay on the computer, how much exercise to do, how far to drive, when to go to bed at night, when and how long to rest during the day, how much media exposure to have, and how long to spend in social situations. Personal rules have an If/Then structure. For example:

- If I've been on the computer for 20 minutes, then it's time to take a break.
- If it's 11 am, then it's time for my morning rest.
- If it's 9 pm, then it's time to start getting ready for bed.

Rules are planned responses, which you use as a substitute for old habitual behaviors. Over time, the new behavior becomes a habit. For more on personal rules, see the previous chapter.

The third aspect focuses on thoughts and involves rewriting our mental scripts. Continuing with the same example, the thought "I've got to finish this job" would be replaced by thoughts such as "If I continue, I'll be forced to spend an hour in bed" or "I'm feeling tired, so I'm going to take a break now." The thoughts you create to counteract the old habit remind you of the consequences of continuing the old ways (increased symptoms) or reinforce the alternative (control).

Part of changing scripts is reframing our view of ourselves to support positive behaviors. For example, one person in our program has changed her view of taking rest breaks. She used to tell herself she was weak for lying down during the day. Now, when she rests her self-talk is, "I am helping myself to be healthy. I am saving energy to spend time with my husband or to baby sit my grandchildren."

The fourth part of habit change is support: having people around us who understand our situations and will support our efforts to change. Getting support may require that we educate the people in our lives about CFS and fibromyalgia. We can also get support from other people with CFS and FM, as well as from counselors.

Index

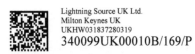

Lightning Source UK Ltd.
Milton Keynes UK
UKHW031837280319
340099UK00010B/169/P